ON-CALL
in
Burns

Angelos Mantelakis
Specialist Trainee in Plastic and Reconstructive Surgery,
West Midlands

Ross Weale
Specialist Trainee,
The Welsh Centre for Burns and Plastic Surgery

Quentin Frew
Consultant Plastics and Burns Surgeon,
St Andrew's Centre for Burns and Plastic Surgery

Medical Illustrations by Gemma Batten

Series editors:
Mr Karl F.B. Payne
Clinical Lecturer in Oral & Maxillofacial Surgery, University of Birmingham
Specialty Trainee in Oral and Maxillofacial Surgery, West Midlands Deanery

Mr Arpan S. Tahim
Honorary Postdoctoral Fellow, UCL Institute of Education

Mr Alexander M.C. Goodson
Oral and Maxillofacial Surgery Consultant, Queen Alexandra Hospital, Portsmouth

First published in 2023 by Libri Publishing

ISBN 978-1-911450-84-9

A CIP catalogue record for this book is available from The British Library

Cover and Design by Carnegie Book Production

Printed in the UK by Halstan

Libri Publishing
Brunel House
Volunteer Way
Faringdon
Oxfordshire
SN7 7YR

Tel: +44 (0)845 873 3837

www.libripublishing.co.uk

CONTENTS

ABOUT THE BOOK EDITORS

Angelos Mantelakis BSc (Hons), MBBS (Lon), MRCS (Eng)

Specialist Trainee in Plastic and Reconstructive Surgery, West Midlands

Ross Weale BSc, MBBS, MRCS (Eng), MSc

Specialist Trainee, The Welsh Centre for Burns and Plastic Surgery

Mr Quentin Frew MBChB, BSc (Hons), PhD, FRCS (Plast)

Consultant Plastics and Burns Surgeon, St Andrew's Centre for Burns and Plastic Surgery

CHAPTER AUTHORS

Andreas Shiatis BSc, MBBS, FRCS (Plast)

Consultant in Plastic and Reconstructive Surgery, Barts Health NHS Trust

Shehab Jabir BSc, MBBS, FRCS (Plast), FEBOPRAS, FEBHS

Consultant in Plastic and Reconstructive Surgery, East and North Hertfordshire NHS Trust

Alexi Nicola MBBCh, MRCS (Eng)

Specialist Trainee in Plastic and Reconstructive Surgery, Thames Valley

Jiaxin Wen BSc, MBBS, MRCS (Eng)

Specialist Trainee in Plastic and Reconstructive Surgery, London

Satyendra Kumar Singh MBBS, MSc (UCL), MRCS (Eng)

Senior Clinical Fellow in Plastic and Reconstructive Surgery, East Midlands

Gemma Louise Batten, MBChB

Junior Clinical Fellow in Plastic and Reconstructive Surgery, London

ABOUT THE EDITORIAL TEAM

Mr Karl F.B. Payne

BMedSci (Hons) BMBS BDS MRCS PhD

Clinical Lecturer in Oral & Maxillofacial Surgery, University of Birmingham

Specialty Trainee in Oral and Maxillofacial Surgery, West Midlands Deanery

Mr Arpan S. Tahim

BSc (Hons) MBBS BDS MRCS MEd PhD

Honorary Postdoctoral Fellow, UCL Institute of Education

Mr Alexander M.C. Goodson

BSc (Hons) FRCS (OMFS) DOHNS

Oral and Maxillofacial Surgery Consultant, Queen Alexandra Hospital, Portsmouth

ABOUT THE ON-CALL SERIES

The 'On-Call' series is a unique learning resource consisting of concise, accessible and highly readable books. Authored and edited by a team with a strong focus on medical and surgical education, they have proven to be highly useful both for junior doctors seeking guidance early on in their clinical rotations and for those with more experience who are looking to consolidate and develop their knowledge. Written as 'survival guides', each book covers common presentations in the emergency, ward and clinic settings, along with a detailed step-by-step description of typical surgical procedures. The attention to hands-on practical advice with easy-to-follow instructions means they are the only handbooks that a junior trainee should not be without.

ABBREVIATIONS

ABG – arterial blood gas
AC – alternating current
ARDS – acute respiratory distress syndrome
ATLS – Advanced Trauma Life Support
BAPRAS – British Association of Plastic, Reconstructive and Aesthetic Surgeons
BOAST – British Orthopaedic Association Standards for Trauma
DC – direct current
ECG – electrocardiogram
ED – emergency department
FBC – full blood count
FFP – fresh frozen plasma
FTSG – full-thickness skin graft
G and S – group and save
GCS – Glasgow Coma Scale
GP – general practitioner
Hb – haemoglobin
HF – hydrofluoric
IO – intraosseous
IV – intravenous
kg – kilogram(s)
LASER – light amplification by stimulated emission of radiation
MDT – multi-disciplinary team
NAI – non-accidental injury
SJS – Stevens–Johnson syndrome
SSSS – staphylococcal scalded skin syndrome
STSG – split-thickness skin graft
TBSA – total body surface area
TEN – toxic epidermal necrolysis
TSS – toxic shock syndrome
U and E – urea and electrolytes
VBG – venous blood gas

INTRODUCTION

Burns is a subspecialty of plastic surgery that manages a broad spectrum of acute thermal, electrical and chemical injuries, usually in the setting of specialised burn centres. Being a subspecialty not encountered during undergraduate and early postgraduate years, this can often result in anxiety prior to starting a job in a burn centre. This book aims to act as a survival guide for junior doctors, introducing you to the key concepts of burn management and burn surgery, and it may be used both as preparation for your new role and as a quick-access guide during your on-calls.

Burn surgery is unique in the way it requires specialised knowledge of burn physiology and an awareness of the variety of specialised tools produced specifically for the specialty. Upon starting a burn rotation, the plethora of unknown types of dressings and intra-operative tools can be daunting. This book is written specifically to aid in the transition. The reader will start by understanding the basic concepts around burn injury, and the natural evolution of the burn. With this in mind, we then introduce the concepts of accurate history taking and the management of minor burns, progressing to major adult and paediatric burn management. Finally, we cover an overview of burn surgery and the duties of the junior doctor on the ward, covering all essential topics you will need before embarking on your rotation.

This book will serve you best if you read it prior to beginning your first job, starting from the very beginning (skin anatomy) and continuing right to the end (the ward). Once you are familiar with all concepts, it can be used on a day-to-day basis as a 'quick-access' guide, with key tips to help and guide you in making the most of your time in the burns centre.

DISCLAIMER

This book is not a textbook, but a survival guide. All content has been written by the authors and is obtained from reliable sources and based on personal experiences. The authors and publisher do not accept responsibility or legal liability for injury or damage to any person as a result of action or refraining from action due to the clinical material within this book. At the time of printing, drug doses contained within this book were correct, but it is the reader's responsibility to check up-to-date manufacturer and drug dose safety guidelines.

CHAPTER 1: ESSENTIALS OF BURNS

SKIN ANATOMY

This chapter provides an overview of the anatomy and function of the skin, which is the cornerstone in burn assessment and management. It will guide your clinical assessment, and it will help you decide which burns should or should not be managed surgically based on their capacity to heal via secondary intention.

The skin is the largest organ in the body, covering its entire external surface, and is continuous with the mucous membranes lining the body's orifices. It exerts multiple vital functions including protection, sensation, temperature control, immunity and endocrine secretions, all of which may be affected in burn injury (see Table 1.1). It is composed of three principal layers: the epidermis, dermis and subcutaneous tissue.

Table 1.1: Functions of the skin

Protection	Against microorganisms, mechanical damage and ultraviolet light
Sensation	1. Meisner receptors: light touch 2. Pacinian corpuscles: deep pressure, vibration 3. Rufinni endings: deep pressure, stretching of collagen fibres 4. Meckel receptors: sustained light touch over the skin 5. Free nerve endings: pain, temperature, light touch
Temperature Control	Thermal regulation via autonomic nervous supply to cutaneous blood vessels
Immunity	Barrier and adaptive immunity
Endocrine	Initiation of Vitamin D production cascade, aromatisation of oestrogens and leptin production

EPIDERMIS

The epidermis is a layer of stratified squamous epithelium that continuously renews itself. It is composed of various cell types. The majority are keratinocytes (90–95%), with the remainder being non-keratinised, including mainly Langerhans cells (role in immune response), melanocytes and Merkel cells (mechanoreceptors). As a perpetually regenerating tissue, the epidermis maintains a relatively constant number of cells and thickness. The basal cells of the epidermis undergo proliferation for replenishment of the lost cell population following injury (e.g. burns) or for physiological replenishment of mutated or damaged cells.

Keratinocytes migrate from the basal layer to the surface of the skin as they undergo keratinisation. The epidermis is commonly divided into four or five layers based on keratinocyte morphology and position (see Figure 1.1).

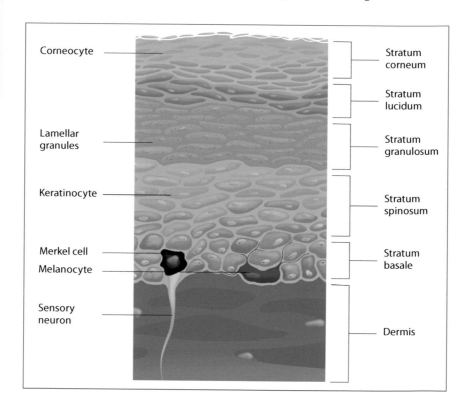

Figure 1.1: Layers of epidermis

THE DERMAL–EPIDERMAL JUNCTION

The boundary between the epidermis and dermis is formed by the basal lamina or basement membrane (BM) which physically separates the two compartments. The function of the dermal–epidermal junction is to provide support for the epidermis, establish direction of cell growth and regulate developmental signals during healing.

DERMIS

The dermis forms the bulk of the skin and is usually <2mm thick (but up to 4mm in some areas, such as the adult back). The dermis serves to protect the body from mechanical injury and houses blood vessels, nerve endings and the epidermal appendages. It interacts with the epidermis in repairing and remodelling the skin during wound healing.

The dermis is comprised primarily of both collagen and elastic fibres, which result in the textural properties of the skin (resistance to mechanical stress combined with glide, stretch and recoil). It has two distinct regional areas: the papillary dermis (superficial) and the reticular dermis (deep) (see Figure 1.2). The papillary dermis lies immediately deep to the epidermis and forms dermal ridges which connect to the epidermal papillae (projections from the epidermis). It is highly vascular and supplies nutrients to the epidermis and plays an important role in thermoregulation.

The reticular dermis forms a thick, dense connective tissue layer which comprises the bulk of the dermis. It contains Ruffini corpuscles (mechanoreceptors), sweat glands, sebaceous glands and the roots of hair follicles. The natural orientation of the reticular fibres in the reticular dermis are termed 'Langer lines', and these are important for wound healing and guiding surgical incisions. Applying traction parallel to Langer lines provides the strongest ultimate tensile strength.

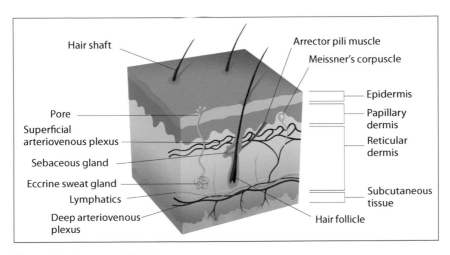

Figure 1.2: Anatomy of the dermis

ESSENTIALS

EPIDERMAL APPENDAGES

These are specialised epithelial structures, connected to the surface epidermis but located mainly within the dermis and hypodermis (subcutaneous fat). They comprise eccrine and apocrine glands and pilosebaceous units (consisting of the hair shaft, hair follicle, the sebaceous gland and the erector pili muscle, which causes the hair to stand during contraction).

During wound healing, keratinocytes originating from the pilosebaceous units, eccrine sweat glands and outer root sheath of the hair follicle migrate towards the wound site and lead to epithelial resurfacing. Partial-thickness wounds that involve the epidermis and partial dermis are able to heal by secondary intention because of intact skin appendages. In contrast, full-thickness wounds with complete destruction of dermis and epidermis heal via the formation of granulation tissue followed by re-epithelialisation from the edges of the wound. Because of the lack of epidermal appendages, densely packed collagen fibres fill the wound site. The ultimate collagen pattern is distinctly different to the reticular pattern found in unwounded dermis, manifesting clinically as cutaneous scarring.

Table 1.2: Epidermal appendages

Epidermal Appendage	Description	Location	Function
Hair follicles	Composed of hair, hair shaft, hair bulb	Most prominent on scalp, pubis, axilla, extremities and face	Thermoregulation, sensation and protection of skin
Sebaceous glands	Exocrine glands	Dermis; predominantly located on the face and scalp	Secretion of sebum (lubricant and waterproof layer of skin and hair)
Eccrine sweat glands	Exocrine glands with secretory ducts opening into sweat pores	Most areas of the body	Secretion of sweat (thermoregulation)
Apocrine sweat glands	Exocrine glands with secretory ducts opening into hair follicles	Mostly in axilla, perineum, areola and external ear	Modified secretions (ear wax, breast milk); no role in thermoregulation
Nails	Composed of the nail plate and nail bed	Fingertips and toes	Protection and allow for grip of small objects

HYPODERMIS (SUBCUTANEOUS FAT)

The hypodermis is composed of lobules of fat separated by fibrous septa, termed panniculus. Collagenous and elastic fibres anchor the dermis to the deep fascia. Considered an endocrine organ, it assists in thermoregulation, energy storage and catalysing the reaction of androstenedione into oestrogen via aromatase enzymes and synthesise leptin (reduces appetite).

BLOOD SUPPLY

The skin is highly vascularised and receives its blood supply via two inter-communicating horizontal plexuses: the superficial or subpapillary plexus (located at the junction of the papillary and reticular dermis) and the deeper plexus (located at the dermis–hypodermis junction). These give rise to terminal capillary loops, each supplying a small unit of skin. Other than arterial supply, these vessels are important for temperature regulation (vasoconstriction results in heat retention and vasodilatation results in heat loss).

NERVES

Nerves to the skin provide both autonomic (vasculature smooth muscle control) and somatic innervation (pain, temperature, light touch, deep pressure, vibration and proprioception).

KEY POINTS

1. The skin is broadly divided into the epidermis, dermis and subcutaneous fat. Based on this, burns are therefore classified based on their depth (affecting the epidermis, part or all of the dermis, or through to subcutaneous fat).

2. Skin healing occurs from the migration of keratinocytes generated in the epidermal appendages. As such, burns that spare the dermis will heal without intervention, whereas deeper burns may require skin transfer (e.g. split-thickness skin grafting).

ESSENTIALS

PATHOPHYSIOLOGY OF BURNS

BACKGROUND

Burns are injuries to the skin and/or other tissues or organs, secondary to heat, cold, chemicals (acid or alkali) or ultraviolet radiation. The most common types of burns are thermal (86%), followed by electrical (4%) and chemical (3%) injuries. Overall, approximately 2% are secondary to assault or abuse, and 1% secondary to self-harm.

Burns result in a cascade of local responses at the site of injury, and if large enough, they can induce a systemic inflammatory response affecting almost every organ system. These need to be considered during the initial assessment in the emergency department (ED), as they will determine your initial investigations and management.

MECHANISMS OF INJURY

Thermal Injury (86% of all burns): Can be broadly classified into three subtypes.

1. *Scalds:* Burn injuries caused by hot liquids or steam. They tend to be superficial dermal burns and are the most common type of burn in the paediatric population (70% of all).

2. *Flame Burns:* Account for the majority of adult burn injuries (50% of all), resulting in deep dermal or full-thickness injuries. They are commonly associated with other concomitant injuries, such as inhalational burns or trauma.

3. *Contact Burns:* Resulting from prolonged contact with a hot surface (e.g. loss of consciousness secondary to epilepsy, drug abuse, or multi-factorial in the elderly) or brief contact with an extremely hot surface.

Electrical Injuries (4% of all burns): An electric current can travel through the body via an 'entry' and an 'exit' point, damaging tissues bounded between the two. Electrical burns can be deceiving, from their apparent small entry and exit points; however, extensive tissue damage can be later identified intra-operatively. The main determinant of degree of tissue damage is voltage, and these types of injuries can be broadly classified into low-voltage (e.g. domestic appliances), high-voltage (usually industrial appliances) and lightning burns.

Chemical Injuries (3% of all burns): These account for a small proportion of all burns but warrant special attention and management, covered in Chapter 3. Common causes include acids (e.g. hydrochloric acid) or alkalis (e.g. cement, ammonia).

Non-Accidental Injuries: Approximately 3–10% of all paediatric burns are the result of non-accidental injury (NAI). This needs to be excluded during the history taking and physical in the ED, and this is covered more extensively in chapters 2 and 3 of this book.

BURN THICKNESS

Burns are classified based on their depth, which is assessed based on several components identified on clinical examination (see Table 1.3). In conjunction with the assessment of burn size, these two factors determine the subsequent management and prognosis of burn patients.

Table 1.3: Burn depth classification

Classification	Tissue Depth	Colour	Blisters	Pain	Capillary Refill	Prognosis (without surgery)
Superficial (epidermal) a.k.a. 1st degree	Epidermis only	Red	No	Yes	+ve	Heals without scarring in 7 days
Superficial Dermal a.k.a. 2nd degree, 2A	Dermis (papillary region)	Pink with swelling	Yes	Yes	+ve	Heal without scarring in 10–14 days
Deep Dermal a.k.a. 2nd degree, 2B	Dermis (reticular region)	Pale (white) or yellow	Yes or No	No	-ve	Heals with scarring in 3–8 weeks
Full thickness a.k.a. 3rd degree	Subcutaneous tissue	White or black (eschar)	No	No	-ve	Heals with scarring >8 weeks
4th degree burns	Exposed or damage to underlying muscle or bone	Exposed or damage to underlying muscle or bone	N/A	N/A	N/A	Loss of burned part

Another description of burns, commonly used in clinical practice, divides them into erythema (epidermal), superficial thickness (superficial dermal), deep dermal and full thickness. It is important to be aware of all these interchangeable terms to communicate effectively with your colleagues.

→ In superficial and superficial dermal burns, the epidermal appendages remain intact and so wounds will heal within two weeks. As such, these injuries do not require surgery.

→ Deep dermal and full-thickness burns result in loss of epidermal appendages which results in prolonged healing times (3–8 weeks). This will likely lead to abnormal scarring (keloid or hypertrophic) with debilitating contractures. Excision and skin grafting is advised in the majority of these injuries.

In reality, burns evolve in the first 24–72 hours (see Chapter 1: Local Response to Burn Injury). At the same time, patients often present with a mixed depth injury (e.g. predominantly deep dermal thickness burns with patchy areas of full-thickness injury). As such, patients require accurate and repeated assessments with clear documentation (see Figure 1.3).

ESSENTIALS

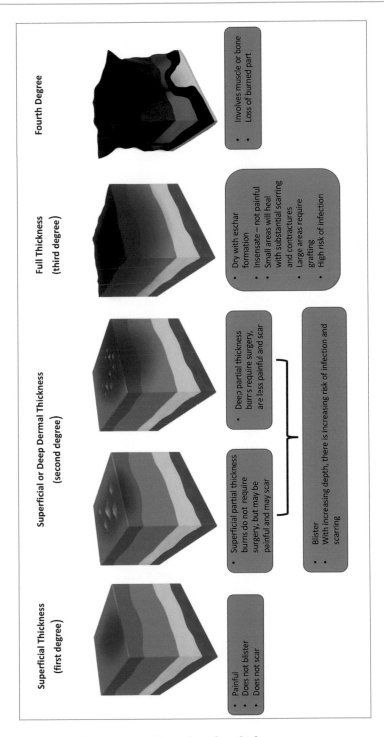

Figure 1.3: Classification of burns based on thickness

ESSENTIALS

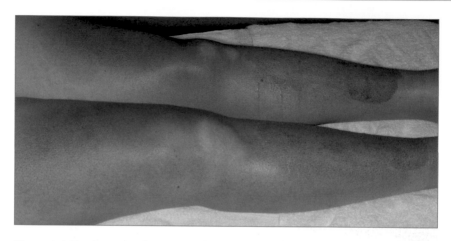

Figure 1.4: Erythema (epidermal burn)

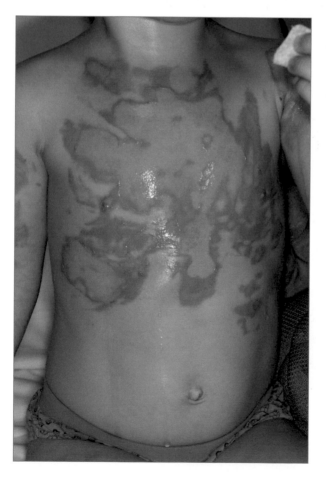

Figure 1.5: Superficial partial-thickness (superficial dermal) burn as a result of a scald in a child

ESSENTIALS

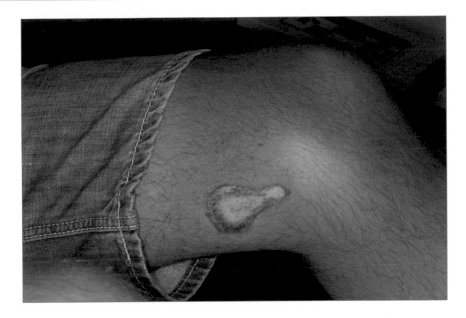

Figure 1.6: Deep dermal burn. Note the 'cherry red' and pale appearance on the deeper areas of the burn wound.

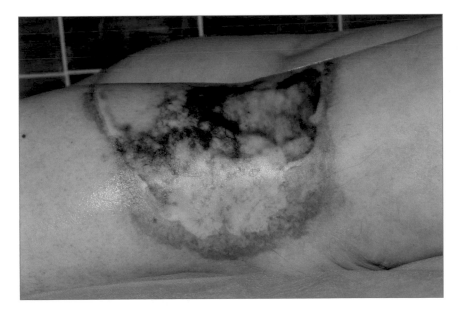

Figure 1.7: Full-thickness burn

ESSENTIALS

LOCAL RESPONSE TO BURN INJURY

Burn injury results in coagulative necrosis (i.e. structural necrosis) of the different layers of the skin and underlying tissues. At the site of cutaneous burns, three concentric zones of injury are typically formed (described by Jackson in 1947):

1. **Zone of Coagulation:** Most central zone, at the point of maximum damage. This area is characterised by irreversible tissue loss secondary to established coagulative necrosis and coagulated blood vessels.

2. **Zone of Stasis:** Represents an area of ischaemia coupled with static blood flow. This zone has the potential to progress to permanent tissue loss, or to heal if tissue perfusion is increased. Adequate resuscitation, cooling, prevention of infection and adequate wound care would result in tissue recovery.

3. **Zone of Hyperaemia:** Most peripheral zone, characterised by resultant peripheral vasodilatation and increased blood flow. This area will recover, unless there is severe systemic insult (e.g. severe sepsis or prolonged hypotension with hypoperfusion).

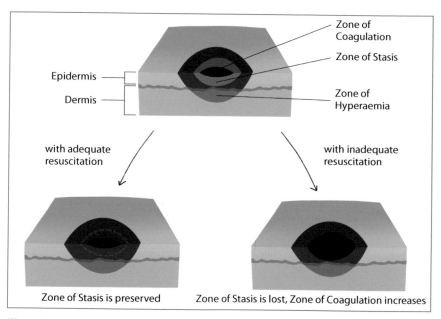

Figure 1.8: Zones of injury and potential outcomes of progression within 24–48 hours. Note that sometimes the initial burn may expand in area and depth. Appropriate first aid in the early stages may salvage the zone of stasis and may make the difference between managing a burn conservatively versus requiring surgical excision and skin grafting.

SYSTEMIC RESPONSE TO BURN INJURY

Once a burn affects 30% of the total body surface area (TBSA), inflammatory cytokines and mediators are released and enter the circulation, resulting in systemic consequences affecting virtually every organ system in the body. These, coupled with effects of the local response to injury, can result in life-threatening organ dysfunction and are the prime drivers of morbidity and mortality in major burn patients. The most serious injuries following a major burn (often referred to as a 'resuscitation burn') are outlined in Table 1.4, and these should be considered during the initial assessment in the ED as well as in the subsequent inpatient management.

In clinical practice, any burns >15% TBSA in adults or >10% in children are treated as resuscitation burns, due to their potential for a severe systemic response to the injury.

Table 1.4: Potential consequences of major burns per organ system

System Affected	Local Injury Pattern	Systemic Injury Pattern
Respiratory system	• Inhalation of hot gases resulting in oedema and airway obstruction • Carbon Monoxide (CO) poisoning (treat with high-flow Oxygen 100%, for 48 hours) • Circumferential chest burns may restrict respiration mandating an escharotomy	• Bronchoconstriction • Acute respiratory distress syndrome (ARDS) – carries 26–40% mortality rate, requires ITU admission and management • Other: pulmonary oedema secondary to over-hydration, supra-added infection
Cardiovascular system	Systemic hypotension and end-organ hypoperfusion secondary to • Vasodilation and increased vascular permeability; leading to loss of proteins to the interstitial compartment (hypo-albuminaemia) and oedema • Hypovolaemia and shock from fluid losses and/or sepsis • Decreased myocardial contractility	
Renal system	Acute kidney injury (AKI) secondary to hypovolaemia, sepsis and/or rhabdomyolysis	

System Affected	Local Injury Pattern	Systemic Injury Pattern
Metabolic system	• Hypothermia secondary to loss of skin	• Increased metabolic rate by up to 3x, necessitates early and aggressive enteral feeding • Electrolyte disturbances (hyperkalaemia, hypocalcaemia, and hyper- or hypo-natremia)
Musculoskeletal system	Circumferential burns may result in compartment syndrome mandating an escharotomy	Oedema and fluid overload may result in compartment syndrome mandating a fasciotomy
Gastro-intestinal system	Acute peptic stress ulceration (Curling's ulcers)	
Immunological system	• Downregulation of the innate and adaptive immune responses • Systemic inflammatory response syndrome • Sepsis	
Haematological system	• Disseminated intravascular coagulopathy • Haemolysis secondary to red-blood-cell damage from heat or angiopathy (resulting in low Hb)	

KEY POINTS

1. Burns are complex injuries resulting in both local and systemic consequences.

2. Basic knowledge of the underlying pathophysiology and body responses to burns is essential and will guide your initial assessment, investigations, treatment and subsequent monitoring of your patients.

3. Different types of burn will lead to different injury patterns, which may require different management. These will be addressed separately under the management section.

4. Approximately 6.5% of all burned patients receive treatment in specialised burn centres.

CHAPTER 2: ASSESSMENT OF BURNS

HISTORY TAKING FOR BURNS

It's important to adapt your history taking to each patient, and for each mechanism of burn. Bear in mind that this may be the only time you are able to take a history if intubation is required. Ensure that your documentation is meticulous.

HISTORY OF THE INJURY
- When: Exact date and time of injury
- How: Mechanism of injury
    - Contact, scald, explosion, flash, submersion
- What: Cause of the burn
    - Heat, chemical, electrical, radiation
- How long: Duration of exposure to energy source
- Where: Place of injury
    - Environment
        - Outside: contamination with soil
        - Industrial: chemical contaminants
    - Enclosed space
        - Could carbon monoxide or cyanide poisoning have occurred?
        - Could there be a possibility of an inhalation injury?
- Was clothing worn at time of injury? How many layers? Was clothing removed?
- Who was present at the scene? Can a collateral history be gathered?

Note: The mechanism of a burn may indicate its depth, for example:

- Flash – superficial epidermal

- Scald – superficial epidermal or superficial dermal

- Flame – deep dermal or full thickness

- Contact – deep dermal or full thickness

- Chemical – full thickness

- Electrical – full thickness

A longer duration of exposure to an energy source could result in a burn that is deeper than you suspect – for example, a brief touch to a very warm radiator may cause a little irritation, but to lie unconscious against one for several hours can produce a deep, significant injury.

Table 2.1: Follow-up questions based on the mechanism of injury

Scald	• Time since liquid was boiled • What was the liquid? (oil, food) • Any additives (e.g. sugar and milk, especially given that most scalds are caused by tea or coffee) • Volume of liquid
Electrical Injuries	• Have entrance and exit sites been identified? • Was the voltage domestic or industrial (DC or AC)? • Was there visible arcing or a flash? • What was the contact time? • Was the patient's clothing ignited? • Was there any loss of consciousness? • Was the patient 'thrown' any distance away? • Were there any immediate symptoms post-event? (e.g. palpitations, shaking or seizing)

| Chemical | • Chemical agent
    • Alkalis (e.g. cement, fertiliser)
    • Acids
• Physical form
    • Liquid, powder
• Has the patient brought the label of product?
• Duration of exposure to chemical
• Volume of agent
• Was a neutralising agent used?
• Was this an occupational incident? If it was, was any protective gear worn/provided?
• If non-accidental:
    • Circumstances surrounding incident if acid attack
    • Police involvement
    • Dangerous substances and unsupervised children (e.g. drug manufacturing in family home) |
| Explosion | • Cause of explosion
• What was the patient's proximity to the explosion? |

ASSESSMENT OF BURNS

Sequence of Events from Time of Injury until Presentation to ED
- First aid received and duration of first aid
    - All burns should receive first aid, defined as cooling of the burned area with mildly cold water (15°C) for 20 minutes, within the first 2–3 hours following the injury. This may reduce burn depth by up to 25%.
    - What did you do after the burn happened?
    - Did you perform any cooling of the burn? If so, how was this performed?
    - How long was cooling applied for?
- Treatment given so far
    - If fluids given, when and how much?
    - If irrigated, for how long and how much?

Systems Review
- Any other injuries possible?
    - E.g. fall from height, road-traffic collision, explosion (think projectiles and blast)
- Were alcohol or drugs involved?
    - Alcohol consumption potentiates post-burn remote organ damage and worsens outcome

- Concomitant alcohol and drug use may predispose towards more severe burns with an increased risk of sepsis and death
- Could another medical event have preceded the burn?
  - E.g. seizure, MI, syncope
- Could the burn be related to self-harm?
- If vulnerable person or child, complete a risk assessment as per your hospital guidelines

Patient Details
- Past medical history
  - Any conditions that pre-dispose to infection
    - Diabetes
  - Any pre-existing cardiac, liver or lung disease
    - Asthma
  - Coagulation disorders
  - Psychiatric history
    - Past surgical history (e.g. splenectomy)
- Medications, allergies and vaccination history
  - Immunosuppression
- Social history, especially smoking

Non-Accidental Injury

The incidence of non-accidental burns in children is estimated to be around 9.7%, with 2% of paediatric admissions to burns units being as a result of NAI. Try to separate the potential victim from any accompanying people in order to gather an independent history and ask more sensitive questions. Consider the need for a chaperone. Although more common in children and vulnerable adults, consider this in all burn referrals.

Indicators for NAI
- Child/patient brought in by unrelated adult/carer
- Delayed presentation with inadequate explanation
- History and burn not consistent with injury
- History incompatible with developmental age
- Mechanism of burn out of keeping with history described
- Pattern of injury
  - Injury to posterior trunk, perineum, buttocks or genitalia

- Burns to head, neck, anterior trunk, upper extremities and feet are more commonly caused by accidents
- Mirror-image injury to the extremities; bilateral burn symmetry implies forced immersion
- Injuries involving the left side of patient
- Deliberate contact burn
- Cigarette burns
- Unrelated other injuries
  - Bruises, fractures
- Parental drug/alcohol use
- Previous history of NAI of patient or siblings
- Inappropriate parental/carer affect or inappropriate affect of the child

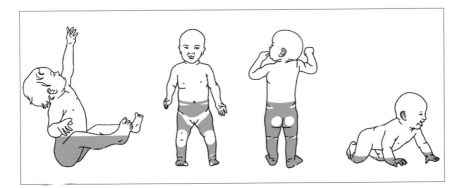

Figure 2.1: Various patterns of forced immersion in babies and in toddlers

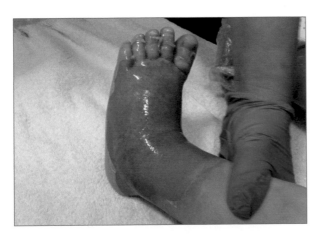

Figure 2.2: Note the pattern of burn injury – well demarcated to the level of the ankle with sparing of the soles, indicating forced immersion in hot water

ASSESSMENT OF BURNS

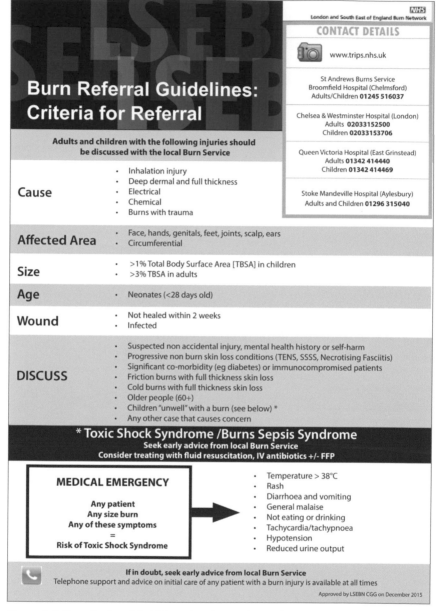

Figure 2.3: Burn Referral Guidelines for the London and South East of England Burns Network ©

INVESTIGATIONS FOR BURNS

The decision for investigations should be judged on an individual patient basis. For the majority of minor, stable burns, patients usually would not require an invasive workup. Nevertheless, major burns can often lead to high morbidity and mortality due to the multiple organ systems being affected. As a result, care is required to identify these early and treat them accordingly. Here follows a list of investigations that may be considered when approaching certain burns patients.

AIRWAY AND BREATHING

Bronchoscopy
- Should be considered in all cases where inhalation injury is suspected. Examples include evidence of facial burns, or if the burn occurred within an enclosed space.
- Bronchoscopy is the gold standard and the most reliable way of diagnosing an inhalation injury.
- It permits direct, real-time visualisation of both supraglottic and subglottic structures. Therefore, upon assessment of the damaged airway tissues, the involved clinicians can make a more informed judgement on the need for intubation.
- Characteristic findings of inhalation injury can include carbonaceous debris below the vocal cords, hyperaemia, mucosal oedema and ulceration.
- Bronchoscopy can also have a therapeutic function, which is the direct removal of foreign material and bronchoalveolar lavage (BAL). The washout out fluid can be sent for microscopy and culture.

> **TIPS**
>
> - Emergency bronchoscopy and BAL for inhalational burn injuries are usually performed in either a burns unit or centre by a burns-trained anaesthetist or intensivist. Hence early communication with these team members in cases of suspected inhalation injury is crucial.

Chest Radiograph
- This is often requested as a part of the Advanced Trauma Life Support (ATLS) assessment.

ASSESSMENT OF BURNS

- Burns patients are unlikely to exhibit chest pathologies at the very early stages of their injury.
- However, it may be requested to rule out other conditions which may have led to or resulted from the initial mechanism of injury.
- Serial CXR may be beneficial for suspected inhalation injuries. The first CXR can serve as a baseline for the patient. At later stages, it may show the development of diffuse atelectasis, pulmonary oedema or bronchopneumonia.

Arterial Blood Gas (ABG)

- An ABG is crucial in patients with large burns, especially those with a high likelihood of inhalation injury. Furthermore, an ABG would be preferable to a venous gas sample as it enables a more accurate assessment of the patient's acid–base imbalances.
- This should be considered in patients with suspected airway compromise/injury or restrictive burns, and in those who are haemodynamically unstable.
- Arterial hypoxaemia is an indicator for inhalation injury. This should thus be suspected until proven otherwise.
- The ABG will also evaluate base deficits, lactate and carbon monoxide exposure. These all have substantial predictive value for the amount of resuscitation required.

TIPS

- Serial arterial blood gas tests should be performed to highlight trends. Therefore, early consideration of an arterial line may be of benefit to the patient with significant burns.

- Persistent metabolic acidosis may be secondary to cyanide poisoning.

Carboxyhaemoglobin

- Carboxyhaemoglobin levels are shown on an ABG and are vital in diagnosing carbon monoxide poisoning.
- It should be performed in all inhalation injuries and injuries that occurred within an enclosed space.
- Increased levels of carboxyhaemoglobin have a stepwise pattern of severity on mental cognition: 15–20% can lead to headache and confusion; up to 40% may lead to hallucination and ataxia; levels of more than 60% are often fatal and result in high mortality.

TIPS

- Pulse oximeter monitoring can be misleadingly normal in patients with severe CO poisoning, so it is pivotal to confirm carboxyhaemoglobin levels in suspected inhalational injuries.

- Levels up to 10% can be found in smokers. This would be normal for them and may not indicate carbon monoxide poisoning.

- Patients are usually already on high-flow oxygen therapy via a non-rebreathe mask during transfer and therefore may normalise CO levels by the time of an ABG.

ASSESSMENT OF BURNS

Cyanide Levels
- Investigation for cyanide levels is not readily available in most centres and is usually time-consuming.
- Cyanide poisoning should be suspected in all burns within an enclosed space.
- Factors that can be characteristic of cyanide poisoning are lactate above 7mmol/litre, persistently elevated anion gap acidosis and reduced arteriovenous oxygen gradient.
- Cyanide can distribute in the body within seconds, and mortality can ensue within minutes. Even upon survival, it can lead to permanent neurological disability; treatment such as hydroxocobalamin must therefore not be delayed.

TIPS

- Cyanide poisoning involves inhalation of hydrogen cyanide (gaseous form) when incomplete combustion of nitrogen material such as plastic, vinyl, wool or silk has occurred.

CIRCULATION

Bloods
Peripheral blood is taken as part of ATLS protocol.

Table 2.2: Blood tests in burns

Blood Test	Importance
Full blood count	1. Haemoglobin (Hb) levels: patients frequently require blood transfusions secondary to dilution from resuscitation or direct bleeding from escharotomies and burn debridement. 2. Patients will often have raised white-blood-cell counts secondary to the inflammatory response, but this may also indicate infection.
Urea and electrolytes	1. Electrolyte imbalance in major burns patients is prevalent. The most common electrolyte abnormalities are hyponatremia and hyperkalaemia. Key to screen for other electrolytes such as magnesium, calcium and phosphate. 2. Acute kidney injury can affect 25% of patients with burns >20% TBSA. Therefore, it would lead to increased urea and creatinine levels.
Clotting screen	1. This should be obtained for baseline values and in anticipation of possible surgical intervention. 2. Deregulations of the clotting cascade from major burns at later stages can lead to disseminated intravascular coagulation; therefore, close monitoring of these factors is crucial.
Group and save	1. Similarly, this should be obtained in anticipation for possible surgical intervention such as escharotomies or burn debridement.

SPECIAL CONSIDERATIONS: CHEMICAL BURNS

pH Testing with Litmus Paper
- This should be carried out on all chemical burns.
- The litmus paper is placed on the burns wound to obtain a 'colour reading'. This is then compared to the colour scale provided on the container.
- Serial testing of pH should be performed during burn irrigation in the acute setting until the neutralisation of the burn.
- It is crucial to remember to test the eyes separately and consult an ophthalmologist if you have any concerns.

TIPS

- Avoid excessive wetting of the litmus paper as this can wash the colour away.

- If the pH is measured immediately after irrigation, it may show a falsely neutral pH measurement.

- If there is a prolonged period for the litmus paper to dry out, the colour may deepen with time.

- Bear in mind, normal value of skin is approximately pH 4.1–5.8.

SPECIAL CONSIDERATIONS: ELECTRICAL BURNS

ECG

- Electrical burns can often result in rhythm and conduction disturbances.

- There is significant mortality in high-voltage electric injuries, especially in those with pre-existing cardiac co-morbidities.

- Cardiac arrest is either in the form of asystole or ventricular fibrillation.

- The most common abnormalities are sinus tachycardia and nonspecific ST-T segment changes (this can persist for several weeks post-injury).

Creatine Kinase and Urea and Electrolytes

- Compartment syndrome and/or skeletal muscle damage from electrical injury can correlate with high creatine kinase.

- This can lead to rhabdomyolysis, which in turn can lead to acute renal failure, severe electrolyte abnormalities and acid–base disorders.

SPECIAL CONSIDERATIONS: INFECTED BURNS

Swabs and Tissue Samples

- If an infection is suspected, all samples should be taken before the initiation of antibiotics.

- Deep tissue samples are more reliable than superficial swabs.

- Sensitivities usually can take several days. Therefore, treatment should not be delayed, and empirical antibiotics should be given.

ASSESSMENT OF BURNS

Blood Cultures and Inflammatory Markers

- WBC and CRP trend would be helpful indicators of worsening infection.
- Blood cultures should be taken before the initiation of antibiotics. This will provide sensitivities which will result in more targeted treatments.

ADDITIONAL TECHNIQUES

Laser Doppler Imaging

- Studies have shown that even with experienced surgeons, in indeterminate burns the accuracy of depth prediction is only 65–70%.
- This technique is a useful adjunct to clinical assessment of burns, especially where burn depth is not well defined, such as in partial-thickness burns.
- It utilises the doppler technique, where laser light oscillation wave frequency observed is proportional to the tissue perfusion adequacy.
- An accurate estimate of burns depth can better support clinical decisions on dressings care and grafting requirements.

Fluorescein Staining for Corneal Injury

- Corneal damage should be assumed in all facial burns. Therefore, screening for this should be carried out in all patients.
- Fluorescein (orange dye) stains the cornea, limbus and conjunctiva. Then a cobalt-blue light is shone on the eye to detect corneal abrasions. This test can be performed within ward settings.
- However, if the patient remains symptomatic without apparent detection of corneal defects, they should be referred to ophthalmology for further investigations such as slit lamp examination and intraocular pressure measurements.

TIPS:

- Remember to do this early on, as it may become extremely difficult to open the eyelids when the oedema progresses following fluid resuscitation.

CHAPTER 3: MANAGEMENT OF BURNS

INTRODUCTION

This chapter will cover the initial management of the burned patient, broadly classified as minor burns, major burns, paediatric burns and non-thermal burns (electrical, chemical, cold injuries, radiation burns and non-burn-related skin loss). Each of these will be addressed individually alongside a plan of action.

Remember help is always available – **if in doubt, call for help**.

MINOR BURN INJURIES

Minor burns are defined as small, superficial burn injuries that can be treated at the emergency department and followed up in dressings clinic, either locally or through a burns unit's dressings clinic. Superficial to mid-dermal thickness burns <3% TBSA may be suitable for outpatient management. If in doubt, contact your local burns unit to clarify if they can take over the management of the patient.

Superficial Burns (a.k.a. Erythema): Essentially similar to a severe sunburn and can be managed at home. Advise the patient to drink plenty of fluids orally and to moisturise the area using an emollient. Advise analgesia to keep the patient comfortable. Although no dressings are required, aloe vera or a moisturising cream may help with symptomatic relief.

Superficial Partial-Thickness Burns: The majority can be treated conservatively. Treatment is aimed at hastening wound healing (wounds heal faster in a moist environment) and preventing infection. These should heal within two to three weeks (if they do not, initial depth assessment was probably mistaken, and a burns-unit referral is recommended). They are often very painful due to exposed nerve endings and therefore analgesia use is encouraged. Blistering is also very common. De-roofing of the blisters is advisable in ED, followed by a non-adhesive dressing and a referral in a local burns dressings clinic for follow-up.

Deep Dermal Burns: In selected patients, small deep dermal wounds can be managed conservatively. In larger deep dermal burns, or following failure of conservative management after 2–3 weeks, they are typically managed with debridement followed by skin grafting. We advise that you organise follow-up with a burns unit for all deep dermal burns.

Infected Burns: These can vary in terms of severity and have the potential to affect burn progression (an infected superficial dermal wound may progress to a deep dermal or full-thickness injury). Small, infected burns can be treated with oral antibiotics. However, any evidence of surrounding inflammation or systemic infection should be treated with a combination of IV antibiotics with or without surgical excision, either in a local unit or major burns unit, depending on local protocols. In the paediatric population, an infected burn in an unwell child may indicate toxic shock syndrome, which is a surgical emergency (see Chapter 3: Paediatric Burn Management: Toxic Shock Syndrome).

MANAGEMENT
OF BURNS

The Four 'C's

The initial management of all burn injuries can be remembered as the four 'C's.

1. **Cooling:** This is a priority in all burn injuries, big or small. It can be done with tap water irrigation or using normal saline (T=15°C for up to 20 minutes may reduce burn progression by up to 25% if performed within three hours of injury). The aim is to prevent progression of the burn and to reduce pain. Avoid iced water as it results in vasoconstriction and causes burn progression. Do not underestimate the importance of this in any burn injury – it can make the difference between allowing a burn to heal via secondary intention versus requiring burn excision and skin grafting.

2. **Cleaning:** With mild soap and water or an anti-microbial wash.

3. **Covering:** Primary contact layer with a secondary absorbent dressing. Some dressings have these all incorporated. The dressing should be changed at 48 hours to review the burn wound and its progression. These can subsequently be changed every 3–5 days (see Chapter 4).

4. **Comfort:** Ensure adequate analgesia is prescribed, commonly over-the-counter analgesics with or without mild opioids, if needed.

MANAGEMENT OF BURNS

Table 3.1: Follow-up of minor burns
(To be used as a guide only – consult with local guidelines regarding your hospital's follow-up pathways.)

Discharge to GP	Superficial burns (a.k.a. erythema) that are unlikely to need any special dressings and would only need a routine review to ensure all is healing well.
Burns Dressings Clinic	Any superficial partial-thickness burn that is unlikely to need surgical treatment and receive a specialist dressing.
	Review all injuries that might need early surgical treatment and plan accordingly.
Admission Criteria	Minor burn that is either likely to progress or has become infected and requires urgent treatment.

MAJOR BURNS

By definition, a major burn injury can be considered as a burn covering more than 15% of the patient's total body surface area (adults) or 10% in children. These have the potential to release inflammatory cytokines and mediators that enter the circulation and result in systemic consequences, affecting virtually every organ system in the body. It is important that these burns are managed in a multi-disciplinary setting, within the resuscitation bay in ED, and include input from anaesthetics, A&E, burn surgery as well as the trauma team. Each of these patients requires an Advance Trauma Life Support (ATLS) and Emergency Management of the Severe Burn (EMSB) assessment with a primary and secondary survey. Such burns require senior input; thus, we advise involving the senior surgeon as early as possible.

Advice for Working as a Junior Doctor in a Burns Unit

- When a major burn is referred, always alert the burns team, including the on-call burns consultant, anaesthetist and sister in charge, before acceptance of the patient. Critical interventions may need to be performed at the referring unit prior to transfer, and input from a senior clinician with experience in major burns management is essential in such cases.
- If the patient has a large TBSA burn and might require emergency surgery in the form of debridement, escharotomy or fasciotomies on arrival, ensure that the theatre staff are also aware and that the burns theatre is warmed up and ready to accept the patient on arrival.
- Once the patient arrives in the unit, the primary survey should be repeated, and the progress of resuscitation should be reassessed.

PRIMARY SURVEY IN MAJOR BURNS

A – Airway with Cervical Spine Control

Major burns can compromise the airway via:

External Factors: Circumferential burns of the neck leading to oedema and airway compromise.

Internal Factors: Inhalation injuries, which can be classified as:

- *Supraglottic*: mainly due to heat which causes swelling of the upper airway,
- *Infraglottic*: due to the products of combustion causing irritation and swelling of the lower airways,
- *Systemic*: carbon monoxide and cyanide poisoning.

Signs of Inhalation Injury:

- History of flame burn or burns in enclosed space
- Full-thickness burns particularly around the face and neck area
- Singed nasal hair
- Cough with or without carbonaceous sputum or evidence of soot in airway
- Swelling of the oropharynx
- Hoarseness of voice
- Stridor
- Tachypnoea
- Dyspnea

Any patient suspected to have an inhalation injury should have a low threshold of needing an intubation. An airway that is patent on arrival may become oedematous over the following hours, especially following fluid resuscitation. It is therefore vital that such patients are reviewed promptly by an anaesthetist, as early intubation is vital in maintaining the airway and preventing further respiratory trauma, as well as acute respiratory distress syndrome (ARDS).

MANAGEMENT OF BURNS

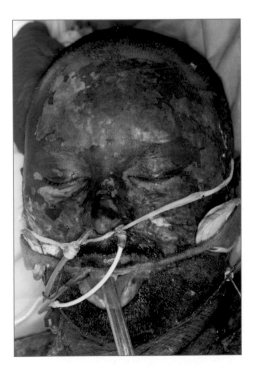

Figure 3.1: Signs or symptoms of inhalational injury should prompt to pre-emptive intubation. This is commonly performed on the scene prior to transfer to a burns centre.

Intubation Considerations

- One should ensure the anaesthetist uses a long/uncut tube because of the impending swelling of the airway. Once intubated, ensure the anaesthetic team keeps the tidal volumes low (<6mmHg) in order to prevent any further barotrauma.

- If properly trained, the anaesthetist might be able to perform a bronchoscopy to confirm the presence of inhalational injury, as well as bronchial lavage to clear the airways.

- Such patients should have serial arterial gas to monitor the pH and lactate.

- Sometimes, patients with large burns may be intubated in the absence of inhalational injury for pain control purposes.

Management of the Airway

1. High-flow O_2
2. Suction
3. Airway manoeuvres and maintenance (including intubation, if required)
4. Consider the use of nebulisers:

   - Salbutamol (bronchodilator)
   - Acetylcysteine (mucolytic)
   - Heparin (can clear casts)

In the case of **carbon monoxide (CO) poisoning**, the oxygen dissociation curve shifts to the left as CO has a higher affinity for deoxyhaemoglobin in comparison to oxygen (up to 240x). Presentation is persistent dyspnea **despite apparently normal saturations**. This is because carboxyhaemoglobin cannot be differentiated from oxyhaemoglobin on light spectrometry, which is utilised in the saturation probe and blood gas analysis.

Cues to the diagnosis on the arterial blood gas include a persistent metabolic acidosis (tissue hypoxia) and increased serum carboxyhaemoglobin levels (COHb). Levels of up to 10–15% COHb may be normal in smokers, but above this level, patients start to experience headache and confusion (15–20%), progression to disorientation (20–40%), syncope, convulsions (40–60%) and death (>60%).

Treatment is with high-flow oxygen for 40 minutes (the half-life of CO is four hours but with high-flow oxygen this is reduced to 40 minutes).

If despite treatment with high-flow oxygen the patient does not improve and continues to have metabolic acidosis, then consider **cyanide poisoning**. Cyanide poisoning is a subglottic injury resulting in loss of consciousness, neurotoxicity and a high possibility of ARDS. It should be suspected in anyone with persistent metabolic acidosis (lactate >7mmol/L), uncorrected anion gap and mentally compromised patient. The treatment for cyanide poisoning is with hydroxocobalamin (CYANOKIT®). Because of its minimal side effects, there should be a low threshold for treatment. This characteristically *turns the patient's urine red*, which may be mistakenly diagnosed as rhabdomyolysis.

B – Breathing

This is assessed by measurement of respiratory rate, saturation and blood gases. A patient's breathing can be compromised due to:

- Mechanical restriction due to full-thickness burns on the chest leading to inadequate ventilation
- Blast injuries related to the burn leading to trauma (e.g. flail chest and pneumothorax)
- Inhalation injury: direct injury to lung parenchyma or systemic poisoning (CO or cyanide).

Mechanical Restriction: A circumferential deep dermal or full-thickness burn affecting the chest may compromise ventilation due to mechanical restriction of chest expansion (eschar is inelastic). Such patients require urgent treatment in the form of escharotomies to correct the restriction (see Chapter 4).

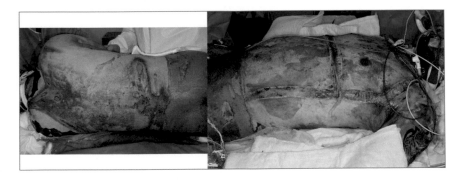

Figure 3.2: Circumferential full-thickness burns may require an urgent escharotomy to improve ventilation.

MANAGEMENT OF BURNS

Blast Injuries: These can be numerous and life-threatening. Examples include flail chest, pneumothorax (simple, tension, open or haemothorax), as well as pulmonary contusions. These should be managed by the trauma team.

Inhalation Injuries: The products of combustion cause direct injury to the lung airways, resulting in bronchoconstriction, as well as direct injury to pneumocytes resulting in inflammation and oedema. At the severe end of this spectrum, ARDS develops. Non-invasive management is with nebulisers (as above) and trial of positive pressure ventilation. If severe, patients may require intubation and ventilation.

C – Circulation

Severe burns result in a systemic inflammatory response syndrome with increased vascular permeability and resultant fluid and electrolyte shifts from the intravascular space to the interstitial space. Early and aggressive fluid resuscitation is essential to maintain end-organ perfusion and to maintain perfusion in the zone of stasis to prevent the burn from deepening.

You need to ensure the following:

1. Each patient should receive IV access via two large-bore cannulas, ideally through unburned skin.

2. At the time of cannula placement, bloods such as FBC, U&Es, clotting, group and save, cross match and an ABG/VBG should be performed.

3. A urinary catheter should be placed to monitor urine output. For any burned patient the urine output should be kept >0.5ml/kg/hr for an adult and >1 for a child. Certain burns (e.g. inhalational injuries or electrical burns) require a urine output of >1ml/kg/hr.

4. There should be early NG tube placement – for decompression of gastric contents +/- feeding as major burn patients very rarely meet their metabolic requirements via oral intake alone. Generally indicated in adult burns >15% (10% for paediatric burns).

MANAGEMENT
OF BURNS

Fluid Resuscitation

Any burn over 15% total body surface area (or >10% in children) requires aggressive fluid resuscitation. The *Parkland formula* is used to calculate the amount of fluid required.

Total Amount of Fluid (ml) = 4ml x Patient's Weight (kg) x % TBSA

Notes:

1. Resuscitation is performed using **Hartmann's solution**.
2. 50% of that amount is administrated in the first eight hours from the **time of injury**. *(Remember to include the amount of fluid given in the ambulance/ED.)*
3. The other 50% of the total volume is administrated within the next 16 hours.
4. Under- or over-resuscitation is often the case. Either can have a detrimental effect on the patient. Remember to titrate the fluid administered to the urine output (>0.5ml/kg/hr or >1ml/kg/hr in special circumstances), as well as the patient's clinical parameters (e.g. volume overload).
5. Complications of under-resuscitation include unstable vital signs, development of acute kidney injury and further end-organ injury. Over-resuscitation may lead to pulmonary oedema, cerebral oedema, ARDS and multi-organ dysfunction.
6. The latest ATLS 10th Edition proposes a modification of the original Parkland formula to avoid fluid overload during resuscitation. This is **Total Amount of Fluid (ml) = 2ml x Patient's Weight (kg) x % TBSA**. In paediatric burns this is 3ml/kg/TBSA and in electrical burns it is 4ml/kg/TBSA. It is important to be aware of both formulas.

MANAGEMENT OF BURNS

Example Utilising the Parkland Formula

A 32-year-old man, weighing 70kg with a 35% TBSA, presents to ED. He was hypotensive so he has been administered 1L of N Saline whilst in the resus bay. The injury occurred at 1pm today, yet he is seen at 3pm.

Total amount of fluid (ml) = 4 x 70 x 35

Total amount of fluid (ml) = **9,800ml**

1. 4,900ml of fluid needs to be given within 8 hours of injury (1pm to 9pm) and the following 4,900ml needs to be given in the following 16 hours (9pm to 1pm the following day).

2. Subtract the amount already prescribed in ED (1,000ml) in the first 8 hours. The remaining volume to be administered is 3,900ml.

3. This remaining 3,900ml needs to be administered between now (3pm) and 8 hours following injury (9pm). As such, prescribe 3,900ml of Hartmann's over the **next 6 hours**.

4. Following this, prescribe 4,900ml Hartmann's from 9pm to 1pm the following day.

Note: The above is **only a guide as an estimate of the volume required for resuscitation**. Factors such as inhalational injury, electrical burns or delay to resuscitation may require higher volumes of fluid to be administered. The response to fluids should always be monitored and titrated to the patient observations, urine output (>0.5ml/kg/hour) and patient parameters (lactate, pH) to adjust for over- or under-resuscitation. The appearance of pigment in the urine may indicate rhabdomyolysis, requiring a urine output of >2ml/kg/hour.

Circumferential Burns and Compartment Syndrome

During your assessment of the circulation, it is vital to examine the neurovascular status of all limbs. As with the chest, the circulation to the extremities might also be compromised due to circumferential burn injuries. Full-thickness circumferential burn injuries should be treated with escharotomies.

In the presence of other concomitant injuries, for example fractures, or high-voltage electrical burns, you must assess the affected limb for signs of compartment syndrome. In those situations, an emergency fasciotomy as opposed to escharotomy is necessary.

Please refer to Chapter 4 for more information on escharotomies and fasciotomies.

D – Disability

The Glasgow Coma Scale (GCS) score should be calculated, understanding that this might be related to neurological compromise due to hypoxic or hypovolaemic shock.

E – Exposure

This is necessary for assessment of both 1) the total body surface area of the burn (TBSA, calculated as a percentage (%) of the patient's total body surface area) and 2) the depth of the burn.

Total Body Surface Area: There are many ways to assess the percentage total body surface area (% TBSA).

1. **Wallace rule of 9s:** This is a tool utilised to assess the TBSA. It provides an estimate of TBSA depending on the location of the burn, calculated as factors of 9. It is slightly modified for its application in children, who have a larger head compared to the rest of the body.

Table 3.2: Wallace rule of 9s

Involved Area	TBSA (%) in Adults	TBSA (%) in Children*
Head	9%	18%
Upper limb (each limb)	9%	9%
Thorax and abdomen	18%	18%
Back	18%	18%
Lower limb (each limb)	18%	14%
Scrotum	1%	N/A
Total	**100%**	**100%**

For children over the age of 1 year, add 0.5% to each leg and subtract 1% from the head.

MANAGEMENT
OF BURNS

MANAGEMENT
OF BURNS

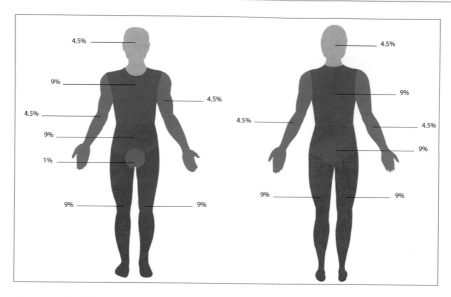

Figure 3.3: Wallace rule of 9s method of assessment of TBSA

2. **Lund and Browder chart:** Utilises the rule of 9s (as shown above) but further helps in a more accurate estimate of % TBSA in paediatric burns. Unlike the Wallace rule of 9s, the Lund and Browder chart takes into consideration the child's age in the relative contribution of % TBSA of each burned part.

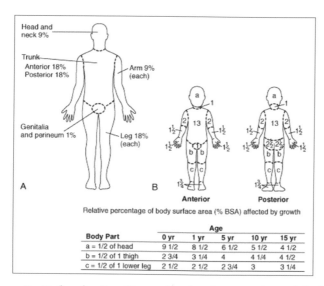

Figure 3.4: Lund and Browder chart for assessment of TBSA

Relative percentage of body surface area (% BSA) affected by growth

Body Part	0 yr	1 yr	5 yr	10 yr	15 yr
a = 1/2 of head	9 1/2	8 1/2	6 1/2	5 1/2	4 1/2
b = 1/2 of 1 thigh	2 3/4	3 1/4	4	4 1/4	4 1/2
c = 1/2 of 1 lower leg	2 1/2	2 1/2	2 3/4	3	3 1/4

3. **Rule of palm:** The patient's palmar surface of the hand corresponds to approximately 1% TBSA. It can be useful in smaller burns to estimate % TBSA.

Burn Depth Assessment: Burns are classified based on their depth thickness, which is assessed based on several components identified on clinical examination outlined in Chapter 2. In conjunction with the assessment of burn size, these two factors determine the subsequent management and prognosis of burn patients.

Ensure you correctly identify and document both % TBSA and the depth of burn (which can be variable – for example, the patient may have an area of deep dermal burn with surrounding superficial-thickness burns). As burns may evolve in the next 48–72 hours, assessments need to be repeated and well documented.

Fluids, Analgesia, Tetanus and Tubes

Ensure the volume of resuscitation fluids is correct according to the Parkland formula based on your final % TBSA assessment following step E of the primary survey (Exposure), performing adjustments as necessary, guided by the urine output. Initial investigations should be reviewed, and the patient should have the appropriate tubes in situ (catheter, arterial lines, NG tube), the placing of which is often performed with the assistance of your intensivist colleagues.

Analgesia is pivotal in the management of burn injuries. Burns tend to be extremely painful injuries, and analgesia is important for patient comfort and for modulating the adverse effects of the stress response to pain. Tetanus prophylaxis should also be administered.

MANAGEMENT OF BURNS

What Next?

1. The primary survey of the burns patients is not complete until we are happy that all the parameters of the ABCDE assessment have been addressed. The key is to be systematic and to address all injuries, not just the burn.
2. Following the primary survey, it is pivotal to perform a thorough **secondary survey**. This is frequently not performed adequately, resulting in delay of diagnosis of concomitant injuries. It should include a thorough history followed by a head-to-toe examination.
3. Eyes should not be forgotten to be assessed, usually with fluorescein dye and a blue light looking for ocular damage. If forgotten, eyes may not be able to be assessed later due to facial swelling. Eye burns are a true ocular emergency that can result in irreversible vision loss, and therefore an urgent ophthalmology opinion should be sort.
4. Clear documentation of the primary and secondary surveys is paramount.

5. Following burn assessment, clean and dress the burn. In the acute setting, cling film is a good dressing option as it promotes a sterile environment, minimises heat loss and pain, and is easy to remove and re-apply. If transfer is to be delayed for longer than 24 hours, a more formal dressing may be required (e.g. jelonet, gauge and bandage).

6. Antibiotics are not recommended in the acute management of burns unless there are signs of infection.

7. A referral to a burns unit often requires a significant amount of information, so have that to hand when making such referrals. Nowadays most burns units require an electronic referral through an online system (e.g. TRIPPS). Images of the burn injury are uploaded to aid the burns unit in assessing the injury as best as possible.

8. Following acceptance, the patient will be transferred to the appropriate regional burns service.

9. If the local burns unit has limited capacity to accept the burns patient, they will contact the national burns bed bureau to find the nearest alternative unit that could accept this patient.

MANAGEMENT
OF BURNS

PAEDIATRIC BURN MANAGEMENT

The principles of burn assessment and management in adults also apply in children. All children should be assessed using a primary and secondary survey, detecting and correcting immediately life-threatening conditions. This section summarises the important differences in the paediatric population.

HISTORY

It is paramount to rule out non-accidental injury (NAI) in all cases of paediatric burns. As mentioned in Chapter 2, any concern for NAI should trigger referral to a major burns unit as often there will be a mechanism in place to investigate and escalate these concerns further.

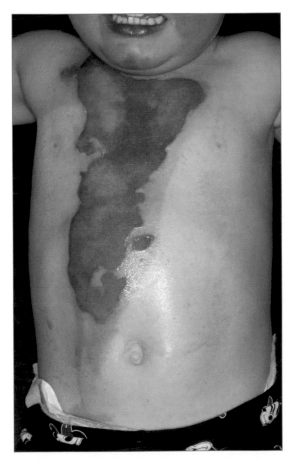

Figure 3.5: Superficial-thickness burn at the torso. This pattern is often caused by accidental scalds incurred as a child tries to pick up a cup of hot drink from a table that is higher than them. This type of injury is common and not typically concerning, as it is not considered to be an indicator of potential NAI.

MANAGEMENT
OF BURNS

PRIMARY SURVEY CONSIDERATIONS

- In contrast to adults, any burn >10% TBSA in children is considered a major burn requiring resuscitation.
- **Fluid Resuscitation**
  - This is performed using the Parkland formula.
  - Additionally to this, children receive their maintenance fluids (given as 5% dextrose and 0.45% NaCl – to prevent hypoglycaemia):
    - 100ml/kg for the first 10kg
    - 50ml/kg for the next 10kg
    - 20ml/kg then after
  - Urine output must be maintained >1ml/kg/hr
  - If extra fluid is required, 5–10ml/kg boluses can be administered.
- **Analgesia:** Analgesia is crucial in the paediatric population.
  - Intranasal diamorphine is routinely used as analgesia in paediatric burns. Diamorphine can only be administrated if a child weighs over 10kg. The dose is 0.1ml/kg. There are specific charts to aid in the preparation of the spray, which is usually prepared by diluting 5mg of diamorphine in a specific volume of saline based on the child's weight. 0.2ml of that solution sprayed in the child's nose will correspond to 0.1ml/kg.
  - o   If need be, intra-osseous (IO) access can also be utilised.
- TBSA in children is best assessed by using the age-adjusted Lund and Browder chart for the paediatric population or the rule of palm. Although there is a modification of the Wallace rule of 9s for children, this is not age-adjusted and is not as accurate.
- Ensure that the child is kept warm. Children are more likely to lose heat than adults due to impaired thermoregulation, larger body-surface-area-to-weight ratio and thinner subcutaneous tissue. Therefore, ensure that the child is never fully exposed when assessing the % TBSA.

SURGERY

- **Surgery:** It will be likely that superficial partial-thickness burns up to approximately 6–8% in children are debrided in theatres and managed with special dressings. These dressings are often used to reduce pain in children and require no dressing changes, in contrast to conventional dressings. These are ***applied under general anaesthetic***, so you should thus enquire if your seniors would like you to starve the patient in preparation.

- o   Biobrane® is the most well-known and common specialist dressing utilised in the paediatric and sometimes adult population. It is an epidermal substitute derived of porcine fibroblasts embedded in a nylon mesh. You need to ensure there are no patient religious or ethical issues.

- o   Epiprotect® is a synthetic epithelium (dermal matrix) that is 100% free from human or animal products. It is commonly utilised for facial burns.

- o   Suprathel® is a synthetic dressing composed of polyglactin. It is heat activated and adheres onto the skin. It prevents entry of bacteria and lets less fluid out, hence creating a slightly acidic environment which is also antimicrobial.

Application of Biobrane®

Indication: Most commonly used in superficial-thickness paediatric burns in a confluent area of >5% TBSA (anything smaller than this can be managed with simple dressings).

Risks: The main risk is infection as this may necessitate an immediate return to theatre. As such, it should not be applied after 24–48 hours of injury, due to the high risk of bacterial colonisation, or in any burns that are deeper than superficial thickness.

Benefits: Biobrane® reduces pain and is less traumatic to the child as it requires fewer dressing changes. (Biobrane® peels off after the skin underneath it has healed, and is atraumatic to the child.)

Procedure

1. Biobrane® should be applied in theatres under general anaesthetic.
2. Clean the burn thoroughly with betadine and normal saline.
3. Open up Biobrane® and identify the side with the label 'THIS SIDE UP'.
4. Apply over the wound under tension and stretch to conform to the wound.
5. There are different methods to anchor the Biobrane® to confirm it is under tension – options include mefix, tissue glue or stapling separate sheets to each other in a 'hem'.
6. On top of the Biobrane®, dress with an absorbent and antimicrobial layer.

Post-operative instructions

1. Post-operative antibiotics are usually required.
2. Change outer dressing in 24–48 hours.
3. Conduct regular checks until Biobrane® has lifted off.

MANAGEMENT OF BURNS

TOXIC SHOCK SYNDROME

Toxic shock syndrome (TSS) is a systemic, toxin-mediated disease produced by some strains of bacteria, most commonly *Staphylococcus aureus* and *Group-A Streptococcus*. In paediatric burns, it has an incidence of 1.5–14%, and if missed and/or untreated, it carries a mortality rate of 15–50%. As such, it is essential to be able to recognise and treat this condition urgently.

TSS can occur in every burn size, and is more often encountered in minor burns. After 24–48 hours following a burn, which is initially sterile, colonisation with potentially toxin-producing strains of *Staph aureus* and *Group-A Strep* occurs. Under the age of five years old, only 30% of children have antibodies against the TSST-1 endotoxin (loss of maternal passive immunity after six months, coupled with a relatively immature immune system).

As such, infection may occur at typically 2–4 days following injury. TSST1 is released into the circulation at high quantities resulting in an over-activation of the immune system and an overwhelming immune response that is destructive to all organ systems. This is termed toxic shock syndrome.

Diagnosis

Any child with fever following a burn injury should be treated as TSS until proven otherwise.

Children typically present with shock, high pyrexia and an erythematous rash, alongside gastro-intestinal and central-nervous-system disturbance. Diagnosis is clinical, and there are several sets of criteria to assist you in the diagnosis (see tables 3.3 and 3.4). Diagnosis can be challenging as TSS may mimic other childhood diseases (e.g. scarlet fever, Kawasaki's disease, Stevens–Johnson syndrome), so a high index of suspicion is required.

Table 3.3: Centers for Disease Control and Prevention (CDC) criteria for diagnosis of TSS

Major Criteria (Need All)	Involvement of Three or More
Temperature >38.9°C	GI: nausea and diarrhoea
Diffuse macular erythroderma rash	Muscular: severe myalgia or CK >2x upper normal limit
Desquamation: 1–2 weeks following the rash	Renal: raised urea or creatinine >2x normal
Hypotension and poor peripheral perfusion	Hepatic: raised bilirubin, ALT, AST
	Haematological: platelets <100 x 10⁹/ L
	CNS: disorientation, altered consciousness
	Mucus membranes: hyperaemia

Table 3.4: MARS BAR score for TSS

Parameter	Score Yes	Score No	Patient Score
Mental State			
Irritable / Drowsy	2	0	
Hypertonic / Floppy	5	0	
Alimentary System			
Diarrhoea	5	0	
Vomiting	2	0	
Abdominal Distension	2	0	
Renal System			
Urine Output < 0.5ml/kg/hour	2	0	
Skin			
Macular rash alone	2	0	
Core temperature > 40°C	3	0	
Rash and temp > 40°C	5	0	

Parameter	Score Yes	Score No	Patient Score
Blood			
Tachycardia	1	0	
Falling Hb < 9	3	0	
Falling Platelet Count	1	0	
Falling WCC < 6.0	5	0	
Appearance			
Clincially unwell / shocked / peripherally shutdown	5	0	
Respiratory System			
Tachypnoea	1	0	

TOTAL of first column ☐   TOTAL of second column ☐

TOTAL OF BOTH COLUMNS   (Max 44)   ☐

Total Score	Action
0 - 9	No treatment
10 - 15	Suspect - close observation - treat (see next page) if scoring increasing
16 - 25	Highly suggestive - Treat (see below)
> 25	Diagnostic - Treat (see below)

MANAGEMENT OF BURNS

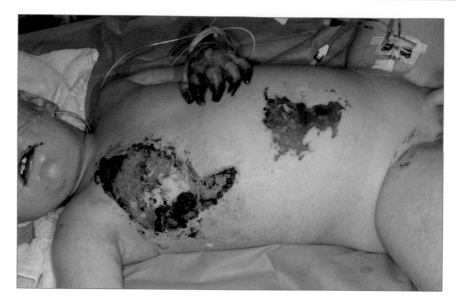

Figure 3.6: Toxic shock syndrome in a child in ITU. Early recognition and treatment are crucial, as mortality rates can be as high as 50%.

Investigations

Bedside investigations:

1. Bloods tests including inflammatory markers, blood cultures and lactate (from an arterial or venous blood gas)
2. Culture swab of the wound
3. TSST-1 toxin for confirmation of the diagnosis (This will take weeks to be analysed, often after the child has recovered, so will not change your management in the acute setting.)

Management

TSS is commonly managed in the paediatric high dependency or intensive care unit. It is important to involve the ITU team, paediatricians and burn consultant early in these patients.

Treatment is based on the following four main pillars:

1. A–E resuscitation, with or without inotrope support, in a high dependency or critical care unit.
2. IV anti-staphylococcal and anti-streptococcal antibiotics, according to the hospital's protocol and/or discussion with the microbiologist on-call (e.g. flucloxacillin with gentamycin). Clindamycin can be added if

needed for a period of 48 hours in unwell patients for its dampening effect on exotoxins.

3. Inspection, cleaning and debridement of the wound. This may be a simple clean and application of an active dressing under intranasal analgesia, or may require surgical excision under general anaesthetic to reduce the bacterial colonisation.

4. Administration of passive immunity against TSST-1 (used in severe cases of TSS; will require discussion with burns consultant and/or intensivist). This is commonly performed via IV IgG immunoglobulins. Some centres utilise fresh frozen plasma (FFP), as this has a 75% chance of containing TSST-1 specific immunoglobulins. However, this needs to be weighed against the risk of blood transfusions.

MANAGEMENT
OF BURNS

ELECTRICAL BURNS

Electrical burns are tissue injury produced from an exposure to supraphysiologic electoral currents or forces. The extent of the injury is dependent on the voltage, type of current and contact period. These have been broadly classified based on the voltage of the current.

Low voltage: Low-voltage injuries are caused by an electric current of up to and including 1,000 volts. These often occur in a domestic setting as UK electricity supply is 240V 50Hz alternating current (AC).

High voltage: High-voltage injuries are caused by electric currents above 1,000 volts. However, usually these are caused by a voltage in the order of 11,000–33,000 volts, as this is what tends to be found in high-tension electricity transmission lines. People working in power stations are at risk of exposure to, or injury from, even higher voltages.

Lightning: A lightning strike usually carries a bolt of direct current (DC) of extremely high amperage, in the order of ten to hundreds of thousands of amperes, and a voltage in the range of a million volts or higher. These make a very distinct injury pattern called arborisation.

Table 3.5: Comparison between lightning, high-voltage and low-voltage electrical injuries

	Lightning	High Voltage	Low Voltage
Type of Current	DC	DC/AC	Usually AC
Voltage (volts)	>1,000,000	>1,000	Usually <600
Current (amperes)	>200,000	>1,000	<240
Contact Period	1–2 milli seconds	Brief	Prolonged
Cardiac Arrest	Asystole	Ventricular fibrillation	Ventricular fibrillation
Respiratory Arrest	Central nervous system injury to medulla	Indirect trauma/tetanic contractions of respiratory muscles	Tetanic contractions of respiratory muscles

	Lightning	High Voltage	Low Voltage
Muscle Contraction	Single	DC: single; AC: tetanic	Tetanic
Rhabdomyolysis	Uncommon	Very common	Common
Associated Burn Injuries	Rare, superficial, Licthtenburg pattern	Common, deep	Usually superficial
Blast Injuries	Blast effect	Shock wave, muscle contraction, fall	Fall (uncommon)
Acute Mortality	Very high	Moderate	Low

MANAGEMENT OF BURNS

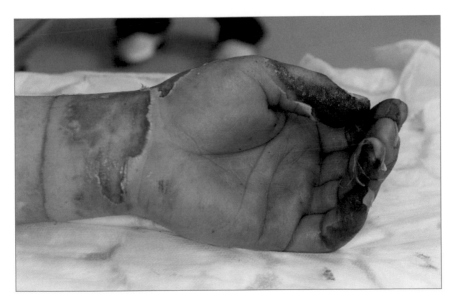

Figure 3.7: Electrical burns often result in small, deep cutaneous burns and are associated with deep muscle injury.

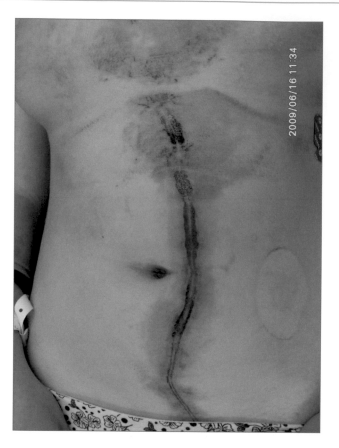

Figure 3.8: Lightning burn pattern in a paediatric patient

PRINCIPLES OF ASSESSMENT AND MANAGEMENT OF ELECTRICAL BURNS

Injury from electrical burns is often multi-factorial. Electrical burn injuries can result from passage of current flow (current transmission) with or without a degree of arc flash (current not passing through the victim but contacted through air or the earth). In some cases, the current or arc can ignite clothing, resulting in the concurrent presence of a thermal burn. In high-voltage injuries, victims may also be thrown back from violent muscle contractions or an explosion, adding in an element of acute blunt trauma.

Electrical injuries are peculiar in their presentation, as often apparent small cutaneous burns may have extensive underlying soft-tissue injury. The reason is that heat production following an electrical injury depends on the differential tissue resistance. Bone and skin pose the highest resistance, producing maximum heat and leading to extensive damage in nearby muscle, blood vessels and nerves.

After an initial history of the events taken according to Chapter 2: Assessment of Burns, patients require a full primary and secondary survey. It is important during your assessment to identify the 'entry' and 'exit' wounds. These can give you an indication as to where underlying injury may be present. In some patients, there can be multiple contact points, in which case these need to be documented clearly.

Electrical burns should be referred to the regional burns services. Important aspects of the management of these injuries involve:

1. Exclude any life-threatening trauma injuries according to Advanced Trauma Life Support (ATLS). Advanced imaging such as CT trauma series may also be indicated and should be discussed with the trauma team.

2. Cardiac complications such as transient arrhythmias or cardiac arrest can occur, although these are rare in low-voltage injuries. All patients must therefore have a 12-lead ECG on arrival. Patients following high-voltage electrical injuries, presence of loss of consciousness or rhythm abnormalities in the initial 12-lead ECG require ongoing continuous cardiac monitor for at least 24 hours. Discussion with cardiology is pivotal in the management of arrhythmias.

3. Extensive muscle damage and swelling put these patients at high risk of developing compartment syndrome, requiring continuous and ongoing clinical monitoring. If the patient is unconscious, intra-compartmental pressure monitoring may be useful. This can be performed by utilising an intra-compartmental pressure monitor system (e.g. Stryker®) or, if unavailable, using an arterial line setup.

4. Muscle injury can result in extensive myonecrosis, rhabdomyolysis and acute renal failure. It is important to monitor for pigment in the urine, as well as creatine kinase (CK) levels. Signs of rhabdomyolysis should be managed with adequate hydration, aiming for an hourly urine output of 1–2ml/kg/hour (75–100ml/hr). Other adjuncts, such as mannitol or urinary alkalisation using bicarbonate, should be discussed with the intensive care team on a case-by-case basis.

5. Management of the cutaneous burn follows the principles of thermal burns.

6. **Indications for surgery:**
   a. Any life-threatening traumatic injury (e.g. intra-abdominal bleeding)
   b. Fasciotomy for compartment syndrome
   c. Escharotomy in circumferential full-thickness cutaneous burns
   d. Excision and grafting of cutaneous burns, as indicated.

MANAGEMENT OF BURNS

CHEMICAL BURNS

Chemical burn injuries are usually work related and account for less than 5% of burn admissions. These can be further subclassified into two main categories: alkali burns and acid burns.

Alkali Burns

Alkaline agents with pH more than 11 produce liquefactive necrosis and therefore result in deeper tissue injuries. Common alkaline products causing burn injuries are cement, phosphorous, bitumen and tar.

Cement: Cement burns are one of the most common chemical burns primarily caused by construction. Due to slow progression, victims sometimes only realise they have the injury after completing the task (i.e. a few hours later).

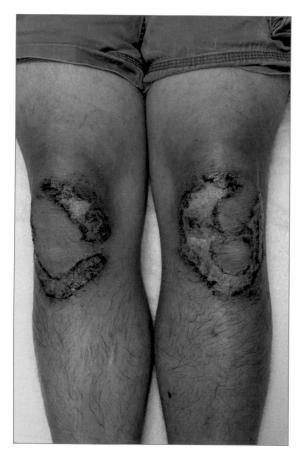

Figure 3.9: Cement burn to a patient's knees. This type of injury is typical of leaning down in cement.

MANAGEMENT OF BURNS

Acid Burns

Acidic agents produce tissue injury by coagulative necrosis. They tend to be very painful. There are numerous products capable of producing acid burns, some of the most common ones include hydrofluoric acid, trichloroacetic acid (found in skin treatments) and acetic acid (used in cooking and cleaning).

Hydrofluoric acid (HF): This is primarily used in etching glass or tiles and in the electronics industries. It is a protoplasmic poison with the potential to cause devastating injuries due to its skin and mucosal surface absorption and rapid onset of action.

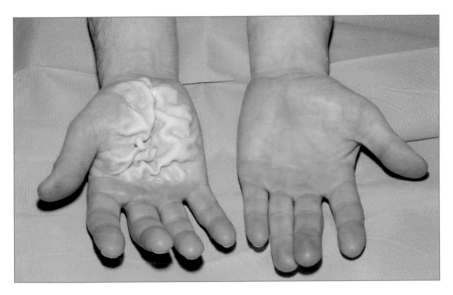

Figure 3.10: Hydrofluoric acid burn to the hand

When encountering a patient with hydrofluoric acid burns, it is important to consider its multi-system effects during your assessment.

1. *Eyes:* It can cause significant ocular burns with destruction of cornea leading to loss of vision. Requires copious irrigation and an urgent ophthalmology assessment.

2. *Lungs:* HF is volatile at room temperature and can thus produce fatal pulmonary oedema and haemorrhage. Assume inhalation in cases of exposure of HF >50%, head or neck burns, soaked clothes and exposure in confined spaces. Involve the anaesthetic and ITU teams early in the management of these cases.

3. *Skin:* Hydrogen (H+) absorption results in extensive tissue destruction and produces severely painful and deep burn injuries.

4. *Electrolytes:* Rapid chelation of calcium +/- magnesium with fluoride ion (F-) results in *hypocalcaemia* and hypomagnesaemia. Significant tissue injury may lead to hyperkalaemia. Therefore, a 12-lead ECG for cardiac monitoring, as well as renal monitoring with serial electrolyte assay, form one of the main pillars in HF exposure management.

PRINCIPLES OF ASSESSMENT AND MANAGEMENT OF CHEMICAL BURNS

Patients should be assessed via a primary and secondary survey to exclude any concomitant life-threatening injuries. Then proceed to take a history, examine and investigate the patients according to the precepts in Chapter 2: Assessment of Burns.

It is imperative to identify the causative corrosive substance as this will aid with your management. Patients may sometimes not be aware what chemical they came in contact with. Clues to this may be found in the history (e.g. glass manufacturing resulting in HF burns), via a collateral history from the employer, or via contacting the national toxicology line for insights. During your examination, a litmus-paper test can direct you as to whether the substance is an acid or an alkali.

Chemical burns should be referred to the regional burns services. Important aspects of the management of these injuries involve:

1. All patients must be assessed with a primary and secondary survey to identify the full extent of the injury and systemic consequences of the burn injury (including inhalational injury from volatile chemicals,

gastro-intestinal effects following ingestion or cardiac dysrhythmias from electrolyte abnormalities).

2. In any chemical burn, it is pivotal to examine for any ocular injury. Protective eyewear is often not worn and so it is common for splash injuries to affect the eyes. Any chemical burn to the eyes is a true ocular emergency and requires prompt irrigation and ophthalmology assessment to perform sight-saving interventions. Irrigation of the eyes can often be uncomfortable, and you should consider using a specialist irrigation set (such as Morgan's lens) or a bag of sterile water with an IV giving set which is set to give continuous irrigation. Some places have access to Diphoterine® delivery washing devices. Avoid rubbing the eyes as this will spread the chemical and worsen the injury.

3. Perform appropriate decontamination, first aid and administration of specific antidotes promptly (see Table 3.6). This is one of the most important steps in the management of these injuries.

4. Management of the cutaneous burn injury is in line with that of thermal injuries. Deeper injuries may require excision and grafting at a later date.

Table 3.6: Initial steps in the management of chemical burns

	Principles	Comments
1.	Stop the burning process	Remove source, clothing, contact lenses and particulate debris.
		Trim fingernails to allow for decontamination and first aid.
2.	Decontamination and first aid	Brush off dry chemical.
		Give copious low-pressure, high-flow showers, avoiding entry into eyes, ear, nose and mouth. These should be started within 10 minutes of contact. This is the most important first step to limit the extent of a developing chemical burn injury. Irrigate until pain settles, aiming for a normal pH. If there is ongoing pain, continue with the irrigation.
		Exceptions:
		Sodium, potassium and lithium burns are highly flammable when in contact with water. Seek advice on the best irrigation technique.

MANAGEMENT OF BURNS

	Principles	Comments
3.	Antidotes*	**Diphoterine®** is a solution which can be used before or after irrigation to chelate both acidic and alkaline substances, reducing their ability to react with body tissues. Can be used for ocular burns. Spray the affected area with a canister of Diphoterine®; continue to spray the area until the canister is empty (this typically takes around 10–15 minutes). In larger burns, or if there is delay in presentation, more than one cannister may be utilised. **Alkali** 1. Phosphorus: Apply copper sulphate following irrigation for removal of particles. 2. Bitumen: Following irrigation, apply paraffin oil for removal – do not attempt to physically remove bitumen. 3. Tar: Following irrigation, remove with Vaseline®. **Acid** 1. HF: Apply 2.5% calcium gluconate gel topically. If pain continues, re-application of gel can be performed. In refractory cases, subcutaneous (SC) and/or intravascular injection of 5–10% calcium gluconate can be considered by an experienced consultant. Monitor serum Ca^{++}, Mg^{++} and K^+ levels and manage electrolyte imbalance. Cardiac monitoring via a 12-lead ECG is pivotal.
4.	Surgery	Sometimes chemical burns, which are refractory to topical treatments with ongoing pain, may warrant early excision to avoid evolution of the wound or to help patient analgesia.

*There are over 2,500 substances that may cause chemical burns. This table outlines the specific management of some of the most common corrosive substances, but you should seek expert advice in all cases.

COLD BURN INJURIES

Cold burn injuries are caused by exposure to extreme cold temperature. Their incidence is increasing due to homelessness, mental health issues, more people exploring winter outdoor activities and industrial exposure. In a quarter of patients, it is self-inflicted.

Extremities are the most affected areas. Cold burn injuries are often small, superficial-thickness burns, but severe cases result in distal limb or digital ischaemia and a requirement for amputation. Cold injuries are classified into two main categories:

1. **Non-freezing cold injury:** Occurs when tissues are exposed to low temperatures (0–15°C) for hours or days. Usually managed conservatively but may lead in the long term to neurological sequalae (paraesthesia or chronic pain) that require ongoing treatment.

2. **Freezing cold injuries (a.k.a. frostbite):** Occurs when tissues are exposed to temperatures below their freezing point, which is below 0.5°C. This leads to direct tissue injury, vasoconstriction and thrombosis, resulting in tissue ischaemia and gangrene. Amputation rates for frostbites have been reported to be as high as 20%, with up to 67% of patients experiencing chronic symptoms related to chronic pain and loss of function.

Patterns of freezing and non-freezing injuries may co-exist in the same limb, although a dominant form of injury will often be apparent. As with thermal burns, these are described according to their thickness and % TBSA, although four-degree classification systems have been described for frostbites to include the degree of ischaemia/gangrene.

Table 3.7: Risk factors for cold injuries

Host Factors	Environmental Factors
Alcohol abuse	Degree of cold temperature
Mental illness	Duration of exposure
Peripheral vascular disease	Homelessness
Peripheral neuropathy	Windchill factor
Malnutrition	Geographical factors such as higher latitudes and altitudes
Chronic illness	
Tobacco use	Contact with conductive materials such as water, ice, metal
Races such as African are at higher risk	

MANAGEMENT OF BURNS

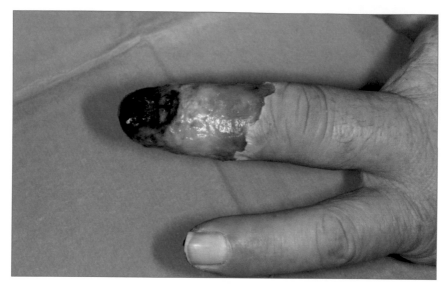

Figure 3.11: Cold injury

PRINCIPLES OF ASSESSMENT AND MANAGEMENT OF COLD INJURIES

1. The early management for all patients begins at the early reversal of hypothermia, and transfer to a place of safety. All patients must be assessed with a primary and a secondary survey to exclude any concomitant injuries, and patients must be rewarmed to normothermia.

2. Once in a hospital setting, commence early rewarming of the affected limb using warm running water at 37–39°C for 30 minutes to 1 hour. This must only take place if the risk of refreezing is eliminated, as cycles of thawing and refreezing result in more extensive tissue injury.

3. Rewarming can be very painful. Adequate analgesia including early NSAIDs (for both pain control and their anti-thrombotic effects), with or without opioids, should be administered, alongside tetanus prophylaxis.

4. All clear (not haemorrhagic) blisters should be debrided to allow for burn depth assessment and dressing management. In severe cold injuries, this may require a general anaesthetic. Apply adhesive and sterile bulky dressings and perform body part elevation. Other adjuncts, including aloe vera (anti-thromboxane effects) and hyperbaric oxygen therapy (improving oxygen delivery in tissues), have been reported in literature, with limited evidence on their effectiveness.

5. In severe frostbite injuries where the limb or digit viability is at risk, urgent imaging in the form of a T^{99} bone scan, magnetic resonance angiography (MRA) or angiography is indicated to assess for degree of occlusion, prior to consideration of systemic thrombolytic therapy (tPA, with heparin to prevent recurrence of thrombosis). This requires discussion with an experienced consultant and the HDU/ITU teams. Repeating angiography every 12–24 hours is recommended to monitor the effectiveness of treatment and determine the cessation of thrombolytic therapy. Improved perfusion following localised or systemic thrombolysis decreases late amputations following frostbite, with maximal efficacy seen when treatment is started within 24–48 hours post injury.

6. As a general rule, cutaneous burns from frostbite injuries are managed conservatively to allow the burn to demarcate, unless the patient develops signs of infection and/or sepsis. The majority are of small % TBSA, and as such even if they develop into full-thickness wounds, they may be managed conservatively.

7. **Indications for surgery:**

    a. Ischemia-reperfusion injury following rewarming resulting in compartment syndrome mandating emergency fasciotomies.

    b. Persistent infection with sepsis refractory to antibiotic therapy.

    c. Amputation of affected digit: amputations can be performed after the wound has demarcated, typically at 6–12 weeks.

    d. Late surgery for reconstruction of amputated part.

MANAGEMENT OF BURNS

RADIATION BURNS

A population with high risk of radiation burn is that of patients undergoing radiotherapy treatments and/or diagnostic radiations. Non-intentional radiation burns are uncommon.

These injuries may evolve with time; therefore, a judicious, watchful wait may be adopted. The treatment for most radiation burns is conservative, including analgesia and non-adherent dressings. Full-thickness wounds may require debridement with skin graft/flap reconstruction and are at higher risk of complications due to a poorly vascularised bed.

Severe radiation injuries presenting with extensive skin damage and multisystemic involvement will need multispecialty intensive care involving intensivist, health physicist, haematologist, reconstructive surgeon and support teams. The initial management should be limited to life-saving measures and supportive treatment.

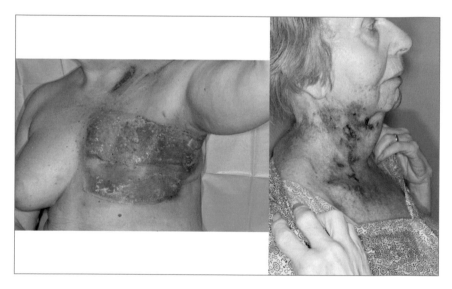

Figure 3.12: Burns following radiotherapy as part of treatment for a) breast cancer and b) head and neck cancer

MANAGEMENT OF BURNS

NON-BURN SKIN LOSS

Burn-like syndromes are rare conditions resulting in non-burn-related cutaneous skin loss that are typically managed in a burns centre. Such conditions include Stevens–Johnson syndrome (SJS), toxic epidermal necrolysis (TEN), staphylococcal scalded skin syndrome (SSSS), erythema multiforme (EM), purpura fulminans, pemphigoid and meningococcal septicaemia skin eruption.

The pathology of most burn-like syndromes is localised to the epidermis–dermis junction, causing epidermal necrosis with subsequent epidermal detachment. The dermis is usually unaffected, and thus cutaneous skin loss from such conditions will not typically require skin grafting.

Stevens–Johnson Syndrome (SJS) and Toxic Epidermal Necrolysis (TEN)

SJS and TEN are potentially fatal conditions characterised by high fever, widespread blistering with cutaneous skin loss and target lesions with mucosal involvement. They are typically caused by adverse drug reactions (phenytoin, allopurinol and non-steroidal anti-inflammatory medications account for 91% of all cases) but can also be idiopathic. The major difference between the two is the extent of cutaneous involvement, with <10% TBSA being termed SJS, while involvement of >30% is diagnosed as TEN (in patients with skin involvement of 10–30%, it is commonly described as SJS/TEN). Mortality rates vary with severity, with SJS having 1–5% mortality rates compared to 25–30% seen in TEN.

The Score of TEN (SCORTEN) is an illness severity score that can be utilised to predict mortality in SJS/TEN patients during the first five days of admission. It assesses the presence of seven individual risk factors that can prognosticate patients on admission.

Table 3.8: SCORTEN for SJS/TEN severity assessment

Risk Factor	1 Point
Age	>40 years
Associated malignancy	Yes
Heart rate (beats/min)	>120
Serum BUN (mg/dL)	>28
Detached or compromised body surface	>10%
Serum bicarbonate (mEq/L)	<20
Serum glucose (mg/dL)	>252

MANAGEMENT OF BURNS

No. of risk factors	Mortality Rate
0–1	3.2%
2	12.1%
3	35.3%
4	58.3%
5 or more	>90%

Staphylococcal Scalded Skin Syndrome (SSSS)

This is caused by the epidermolytic exotoxin that is produced by some strains of *Staphyloccocus*, commonly following localised infection of the upper respiratory tract, ears or conjunctiva. The pathology is limited to the layer between the stratum granulosum and stratum lucidum, resulting in skin erythema followed by severe blistering and skin exfoliation. **Nikolsky's sign**, whereby slight rubbing of the skin results in exfoliation of the outermost epidermal layer, is positive. Mortality rate in children is <5%.

PRINCIPLES OF ASSESSMENT AND MANAGEMENT OF NON-BURN SKIN LOSS

1. There are rare conditions that are best managed in a burns unit with experience in treating patients with non-burn skin loss. Discontinuation of the offending agent, if applicable, should occur immediately.

2. The mainstay of treatment is supportive. This includes fluid resuscitation (aiming for a urine output of >1ml/kg/hr), intravenous antibiotic therapy in the presence of infection, pain control using opioids as necessary, wound care and nutritional support (enteral feeding is preferred, but nasogastric tubes may be required in cases of severe mucosal involvement).

3. Aseptic wound care is pivotal in preventing infection until skin re-epithelialisation, which typically takes two weeks. This is commonly performed utilising conventional dressings. The use of porcine xenograft, allograft skin and synthetic dressings has also been described.

4. Pharmacological agents such as steroids and intravenous immunoglobulins have been described, but there is poor evidence regarding their effectiveness in non-burn skin loss.

MANAGEMENT OF BURNS

CHAPTER 4: PROCEDURES

BURN DRESSINGS

Dressings can be considered as having three components, termed the primary, secondary and tertiary layers. The primary is usually the contact layer, and this may have some active component. The secondary layer is an absorptive layer and tertiary is an outer protective layer which holds the other dressings in place. Some branded dressings combine several of these components so that they can be applied as one dressing.

Table 4.1: Dressings used in burns

Dressing Class	Example	Description and indication	Duration
Primary Layer			
Silicon/non-adhesive	Adaptic®, Mepitel®, Telfa®	Allow for fluid transport across dressing, reducing wound bed injury and pain in dressing changes. Can be used on any wound.	2–7 days but usually determined by other dressings.
Hydrocolloid	DuoDerm®	Active substance that forms a gel when in contact with exudate. Used on low-exudate superficial wounds with no other dressing requirements. Sometimes used around edges of wound to provide a seal for vacuum-assisted closure (VAC) dressings.	2–5 days.

Hydrofibre	Aquacel®	Dressings with good capacity for fluid absorption. Non-infected exudating wounds, good for packing deeper wounds. Aquacel® Ag has silver incorporated into the dressing.	1–3 days, change when saturated.
Anti-microbial – silver dressings	Acticoat silver®, Flamazine®, Urgotul Silver®	Used to reduce colonisation of wounds as they have antimicrobial effects on the wound.	Flamazine® needs daily changes. Other silver dressings can remain 3–7 days depending on specific type.
Antimicrobial – enzymatic	Flaminal®	Consists of antimicrobial enzymes in hydrated alginates. There are two different formulations. Flaminal® Hydro is preferred for low exudative wounds, and Flaminal® Forte for medium to high exudative wounds.	1–4 days, depending on the amount of exudate.
Debriding agents – osmotic	Medihoney®	Medihoney® has antibacterial effects due to acidity, hydrogen peroxide content and osmotic content. The osmotic agents pull water into the eschar, hydrating and softening tissues and thus making it easier to remove.	Medihoney® 2–3 days.

Secondary Layer			
Gauze, Mesoft, EXU-DRY, Gamgee pads		Knitted or woven dressings often used as secondary dressings for fluid absorption. Can reduce sheer at the wound site. Frequently used as secondary dressings for all larger wounds.	1–3 days or until saturated.
Tertiary Layer			
Crepe, bandages		Primary function to keep primary and secondary dressings in place.	1–3 days or until saturated.
Combined Dressings			
Cosmopore®		Soft woven dressing with absorptive pad. Protects wound bed and is gas and liquid permeable. Used for low exudative wounds or post-surgical closure.	1–3 days or until saturated.
Mepilex Border®		Mepitel® combined with an absorbent layer. Mepilex® Ag has silver incorporated in the dressing.	1–3 days or until saturated.

PROCEDURES

BURN EXCISION AND GRAFTING

This chapter provides an overview of the surgical management of burns. It is by no means exhaustive but should introduce the reader to the principles and techniques available, and why they are used. Burns surgery introduces new tools which are not seen in other surgical fields, with new concepts that somebody new to burns surgery may not be familiar with.

The cornerstone of surgical management of burn injuries is burn excision followed by skin grafting. It is indicated in deeper burns (including deep dermal and full-thickness wounds) that are unlikely to heal via secondary intention within three weeks of injury, as this prolonged healing time is associated with higher incidence of adverse scarring (hypertrophic and/or keloid scarring and scar contractures) and infection. By excising the burn and reconstructing with a skin graft, wound healing can be achieved within one week.

BURN EXCISION

Tangential Excision

This is a dermal preserving technique pioneered by Janzekovic, whereby layers of the necrotic surface of the burn are excised down to healthy dermis. By preserving as much healthy dermis as possible, there is an increased compliance of the skin, leading to reduced scar contracture rates and better quality of life for patients compared to total (a.k.a. fascial) excision of a burn. There are various tools used to achieve this, including the Watson knife and the smaller Goulian blade (see Figure 4.1). Alternatively, the VERSAJET system is a high-powered hydrosurgical tool which may be considered when excising superficial partial-thickness burns in anatomically sensitive areas.

With tangential excision, infiltration of fluid containing adrenaline is used to minimise blood loss. There are various preferences for infiltrating a burn before excising. One common formula is to add one ampoule of 1:1,000 adrenaline to a 1,000ml bag of Hartmann's solution. This can be delivered by an infiltration pump or by a pressure bag. Infiltration minimises blood loss and assists in burn excision. Before infiltration is commenced, it is important to mark out areas for debridement, as the vasoconstrictive effect may hinder your burn examination.

PROCEDURES

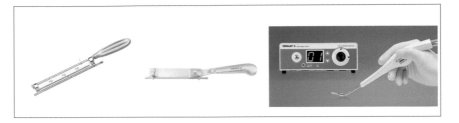

Figure 4.1: The Watson knife, Goulian blade and VERSAJET® system

Fascial Excision

Fascial excision is considered over tangential excision when blood loss needs to be kept to a minimum. This is often for patients with poor physiological reserve or physiological derangement in large catastrophic burns. Fascial excision is quick and minimises blood loss. Commonly performed with monopolar, the eschar can be grasped with forceps or a clip and removed at speed. Haemostasis is easily achieved as the perforating vessels are diathermied. This level of excision leaves unsightly grafts and is therefore reserved only for certain circumstances, as mentioned above.

Within the skin, blood vessels are of a larger calibre the deeper you go. This contrasts with that of multiple punctate bleeders encountered superficially, which are harder to control. An analogy would be to compare the vasculature to that of a tree. By going straight to a fascial excision, the easily identifiable vessels can be stemmed from bleeding, thereby reducing blood loss.

PROCEDURES

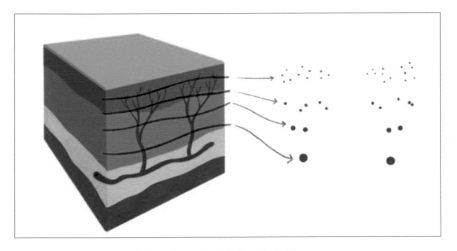

Figure 4.2: Increasing calibre of vessels with depth of skin

Table 4.2: Preparation for surgery

Patient Preparation	1. Review Hb and clotting and correct any derangements. 2. Cross match the patient 2–4 units of blood/platelets and ensure it is ready on the morning of surgery. 3. Starved patient, COVID-19 swab as required. 4. Mark and consent patient (and family). 5. Teamwork is essential: discuss with burns consultant, anaesthetist and nurse in charge.
Theatre Preparation	1. Theatre should be warmed (around 37°C). 2. Request appropriate equipment including tourniquets, adrenaline mix for infiltration, burn excision blades with or without Versajet, a dermatome, dressings.

SKIN GRAFTING

Split-thickness skin grafts (STSG) are commonly used following burn excision due to the large areas requiring reconstruction and the limited availability of full-thickness donor sites. STSGs contain epidermis and a variable portion of dermis, depending on thickness.

Skin grafts are harvested with a dermatome and may be meshed to cover larger areas. It is good practice for the person harvesting the graft to set up the dermatome.

Setting Up the Dermatome

1. Choose the width of the plate depending on what size graft is required. Plate size range from 1 to 4 inches. The blade of the dermatome is applied, which must be done the correct way up (the blade has the words 'INSERT WITH THIS SIDE UP' written on it). Use the screwdriver to screw it in place.

2. Set the thickness on the dermatome. On the side of the dermatome, there is a thickness dial that governs the depth of graft harvest. The thickness dial is in increments of two thousandths of an inch. Common thickness settings include 1 in 8,000 of an inch for adults and 1 in 6,000 for the paediatric population; however, this is extremely variable, based on the surgeon's preference and the depth of the wound following tangential excision.

3. Ensure the dermatome is connected to the air pump and try it before placing it in contact with the skin.

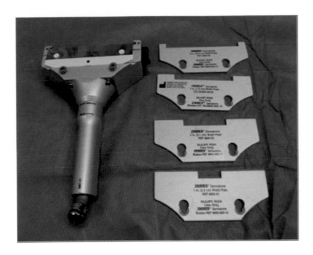

Figure 4.3: A modern-day Zimmer dermatome with the width plates on the right

Taking the Skin Graft

1. Mark area of skin graft using a surgical marker pen.
2. Infiltrate the area to be harvested.
3. The thigh and blade are lubricated with paraffin.
4. Ask your assistant to place tension on the thigh.
5. Using a two-hand technique, drive the dermatome using your dominant hand to take the graft. Use your non-dominant hand to control the direction of the dermatome whilst applying downward pressure.
6. Once the skin graft has been harvested, cover the donor site with adrenaline-soaked gauze.
7. Remove the skin graft with non-toothed forceps and place it dermis-side up on the skin board (skin grafts have a dermis side which is shiny, and an epidermis side which is matte).
8. Mesh the graft as required.
9. Place the graft over the wound (in the appropriate orientation – dermis-side in direct contact with the wound) and secure in place with staples or Vicryl Rapide™.
10. Dress both graft and donor site.

STSGs are commonly meshed to increase the surface area they can cover and allow for drainage of any haematoma which may form underneath. However, the cosmetic appearance of a widely meshed graft is generally poorer when compared to a non-meshed graft.

There are different types of skin graft meshers. Depending on the system, the meshing ratio occurs either by the cutter itself (Zimmer Skin Graft

PROCEDURES

Mesher system) or using a carrier (Meshgraft™ II Tissue Expansion System). In the former, the mesh ratio is written on the side of the cogwheel. In the Expansion system, the mesh ratio is defined by the carrier itself and is written on the base of the carrier.

Grafting Techniques

Generally, burns up to 40% can be excised and grafted using a patient's own skin. Larger burns may need to be temporarily covered following excision, with definitive grafting postponed for three weeks until your donor site heals, whereupon you can regraft.

There are different methods of grafting, each having distinct advantages and disadvantages. Some are outlined below:

1. *Sheet graft*: This is when no meshing is performed, which leaves a superior aesthetic outcome. Can be utilised in areas such as the face or hands.
2. *Meshed graft*: Several degrees of meshing can be utilised to cover large areas (ranging in mesh ration from 2:1 to 4:1).
3. *Sandwich grafting (a.k.a. the Alexander technique)*: For severe, extensive burns, there may be insufficient donor-site tissue to provide enough skin for coverage of the whole defect. To cover these, the Alexander technique ('sandwich' grafting) is commonly utilised. This involves the use of a widely meshed autograft (4:1 or wider) covered with a meshed allograft.
4. *Allograft alone*: This can be used as a temporary solution whilst allowing the donor sites to heal for regrafting.
5. *Dermal matrices*: Examples include Integra®, MatriDerm® and NovoSorb BTM®. Dermal matrices may be used when there are non-graftable wound beds (e.g. exposed bone or tendon) or to increase the compliance of the skin and reduce contracture rates. Their use is restricted due to cost, time for integration (usually more than three weeks), the requirement for a second procedure to graft on the newly formed neodermis and because they have a propensity for infection in burn wounds.
6. *Cell culture*: This describes techniques by which small samples of the patient's skin are harvested, cell lines extracted and delivered back to the patient. These techniques are usually restricted to major burns with limited donor sites.

a. RECELL® is a system by which the harvested cells are processed in theatre and immediately sprayed back onto the patient. This can cover a large area but only provides a small number of cells scattered over the wound surface (i.e. non-confluent).

b. Confluent sheet grafts from cultures require processing in a lab, are fragile and can take 3–4 weeks to be processed.

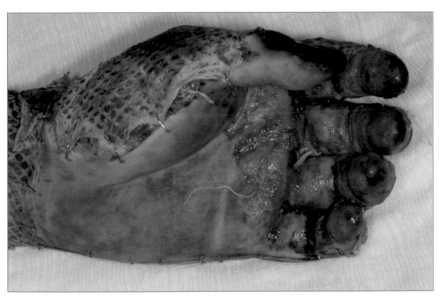

Figure 4.4: Meshed split-thickness skin graft to the hand, secured with staples

PROCEDURES

FINAL NOTE

• There are different schools of thought regarding the timing and type (autograft versus allograft) of grafting in the acute setting, so it is wise to follow the local guidelines and consultant preferences.

ESCHAROTOMY

Full-thickness burns result in the formation of inelastic eschar. In cases of circumferential full-thickness burns, the inelastic eschar does not accommodate for the swelling secondary to tissue injury or fluid resuscitation, leading to progressive vascular compromise (in the limbs) or impaired respiration (trunk). This is a surgical emergency and requires release in a procedure known as escharotomy, which is a surgical incision of the constricting eschar.

Note: This should be performed by a person familiar with this procedure. Although it is an emergency, done incorrectly it may lead to inadvertent bleeding, infection and incomplete release, with ongoing vascular compromise. There may be time to transfer these patients to a burns unit for this to be performed if it cannot be performed locally. Ideally, escharotomies should be performed by a burns specialist in a dedicated burns theatre.

Procedure

1. Use monopolar diathermy to cut through the eschar down to healthy subcutaneous fat, going from:
   a. Proximal to distal
   b. From unburnt skin to unburnt skin (to ensure release of the entire length of the circumferential burn)
   c. Along mid-axial/mid-axillary lines – avoiding any major structures.
2. Ensure adequate release via examining for any restricted areas and return of limb circulation.
3. Ensure adequate haemostasis.
4. Leave wounds open and dress the burn with a non-constrictive dressing.

PROCEDURES

Table 4.3: Escharotomy per anatomical site

Chest	1. Incisions are made in the anterior axillary lines and must be joined by a transverse incision below the costal margin. 2. If the release is incomplete (patient still requiring high ventilatory pressures), the escharotomy can be continued below the clavicles.
Limbs	1. Place the patient in the supine position, with the upper limbs supinated and the lower limbs in the neutral position. 2. Perform 2x incisions (medially and laterally) along the mid-axial lines with curving around important structures (ulnar nerve medially at the elbow, common peroneal nerve laterally at the knee).
Hands	1. 2x incisions dorsally over the 2nd and 4th metacarpals, 2x further incisions over the thenar and hypothenar eminences and a final incision to release the carpal tunnel. 2. Digital escharotomies are sometimes performed.

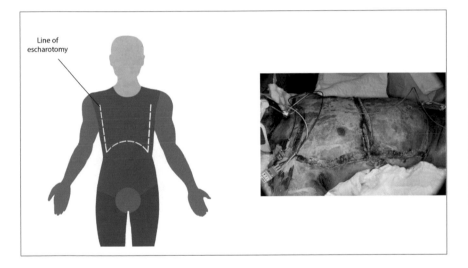

Line of escharotomy

Figure 4.5: Chest escharotomies

PROCEDURES

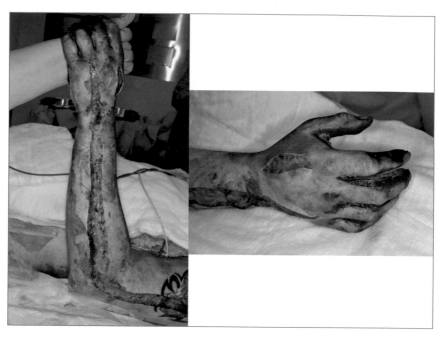

Figure 4.6: Upper-limb and hand escharotomies

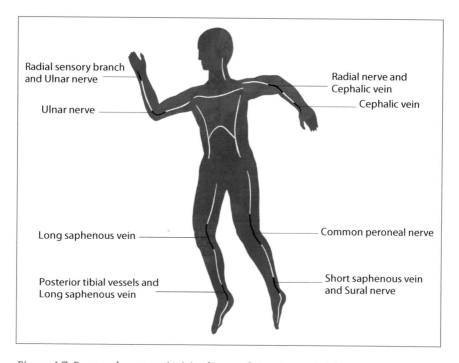

Figure 4.7: Burn escharotomy incision lines and structures at risk

FASCIOTOMY

Fasciotomy is the surgical treatment option for compartment syndrome, which in the realm of burns surgery should be considered in all high-voltage electrical burns. It is distinctly different from an escharotomy. An escharotomy releases the eschar alone, going down to healthy subcutaneous fat, whereas during fasciotomy you are incising the fascia of the muscle compartments to release the pressure from within.

General Principles of a Fasciotomy

1. Best performed under general anaesthetic.
2. Fasciotomy procedure (see Table 4.4):
   a. Ensure adequate release of all muscle compartments.
3. Debridement of devitalised tissues.
4. Leave wound open.
5. Light dressing, elevation.
6. Distal monitoring of adequate perfusion by capillary refill time or aided by pulse oximeter.

PROCEDURES

Table 4.4: Fasciotomy incisions per anatomical site

Lower Limb	1. For UK-based surgeons, the BOAST/BAPRAS guidelines should be consulted. The superficial and deep posterior compartments are decompressed by an incision placed 12–15mm just posterior to the posteromedial border of the tibia, down to 5cm above the medial malleolus. 2. The anterior and lateral (peroneal) compartments are decompressed by an incision 2cm lateral to the crest of the tibia, down to just above the lateral malleolus.
Forearm	1. Incision started between thenar and hypothenar eminences (similar to carpal tunnel incision). At the wrist crease, continue transversely ulnarly to release the Guyon's canal. 2. Next, carry out the incision approximately 5cm proximal to the wrist crease, remaining on the ulnar site to create a flap for median nerve coverage. 3. Then curve the incision radially to reach the radial apex at approximately two-thirds of the way up the forearm. 4. Finally, the incision is curved in the ulnar direction again, up to the radial aspect of the medial epicondyle. (At this point it can be carried upward to explore the brachial artery.) 5. The superficial and deep anterior compartments can be released via this incision. Significant release of the volar compartments decreases the tension on the dorsal compartments, but if significant tension persists, an incision can be made at the mid-point of the dorsal forearm. The mobile wad compartment is released at the apex of radial portion of the incision.
Hands	1. 2x incisions dorsally over the 2nd and 4th metacarpals to release the palmar and dorsal interossei and adductor pollicis (8x compartments). 2. 2x further incisions over the thenar and hypothenar eminences to release the thenar and hypothenar compartments (2x compartments). 1. Final incision at the mid-palm to release the carpal tunnel.

PROCEDURES

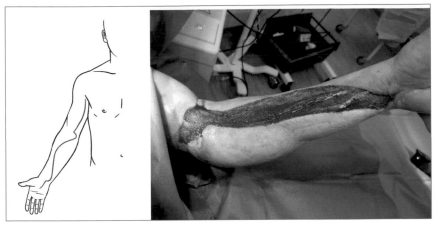

Figure 4.8: Fasciotomy incisions for the forearm. Ensure that all muscle compartments are released and confirm the return of circulation intra-operatively. (Permission for open reuse as per WikiMedia ©.)

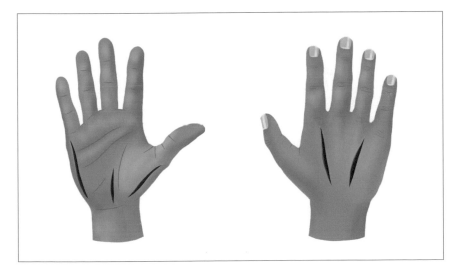

Figure 4.9: Fasciotomy incisions for the hand.

PROCEDURES

BURNS RECONSTRUCTION

With advances in critical care and development of evidence-based guidelines in burn management, survival rates following burns have massively improved over the last 80 years (>90% of burn victims survive). Burn survivors, however, often have debilitating functional and cosmetic sequelae that often require ongoing, long-term management. This has created a new focus on the area of burn reconstruction.

Priorities for reconstruction can be functional (vision, eating, movement and function, or pain) or cosmetic. Prevention remains paramount, and lies in pre-hospital and acute hospital management of the burn. These include the appropriate use of first aid to minimise burn progression, early excision with maximal dermal preservation, the use of thicker grafts and limiting meshed-skin-graft usage. All these topics have been covered in previous chapters of this book.

Ongoing early scar management is pivotal to prevent contractures. Scar maturation takes up to 18 months and ongoing massaging, stretching and appropriate use of splints and pressure garments should start as soon as possible. Whilst waiting for full scar maturation, problematic scars can be managed with non-surgical methods, such as steroids, LASER (many available techniques exist), needling or a combination of these techniques.

Patients often have multiple areas they would like to address during the burn reconstruction process. During initial consultations, the patient is asked to provide a priority list of what is troubling them the most. This is followed by a discussion about what is realistic or what else could be done instead (e.g. release of a shoulder scar first may be preferable in terms of range of motion compared to reconstruction of the hand first), keeping a priority on the functional elements. Non-surgical and surgical options are then discussed with the patient and MDT to reach a final plan of treatment.

Often, patients require multiple operations to address the burn scar sequelae; as such, patient compliance is imperative before offering any surgical procedure. It is commonplace to begin with the most achievable operation, so the patient becomes more comfortable (coming back to a burns unit can be very traumatic for burn victims) and confident in what will be a long journey to reconstruction.

There are numerous techniques utilised in burn reconstruction, ranging from scar releases to local or regional flaps, which are outside of the remit of this survival guide to burns. It is, however, important to understand that burns are not only an acute condition, but can also result in chronic sequalae requiring long-term management.

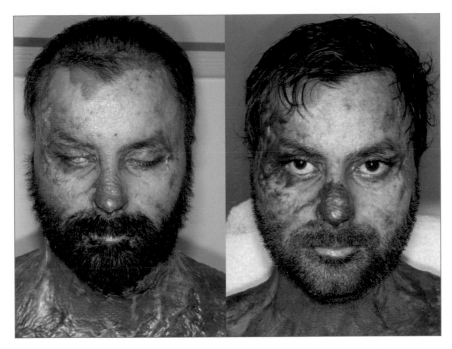

Figure 4.10: With increases in survival of major burn injuries, a focus on quality of life and burns reconstruction is becoming ever more important.

PROCEDURES

CHAPTER 5: THE WARD

Burns is a unique specialty in which management of a patient with burns involves a broad multi-disciplinary team. You need to consider your input from an acute surgical point of view, and how it fits into the whole picture of treating the burned patient.

GENERAL PRINCIPLES: THE TEAM

The importance of burns centres for treatment of patients with burns is largely due to the access they provide to a specialised burns MDT (multi-disciplinary team). It has been well documented that this results in a significant survival benefit. It is shown that there is a lower mortality rate with major burns when treated in a specialist burns ITU compared to patients treated in a critical care setting alone.

To offer the best possible care, it is important to be aware of the teams that are involved in the daily care of a patient with a burn.

- Surgical team
- Intensive care team/anaesthetics
- Microbiology
- Paediatricians
- Burns nursing staff
- Dietitians
- Pain team
- Occupational therapists
- Physiotherapists
- Psychologists/psychiatry
- Social services

There are also multiple other teams such as general surgeons, orthopaedic surgeons, prosthetists, dermatologists, speech and language, and others that may be called on as dictated by the cases.

THE HANDOVER LIST

An up-to-date handover list is pivotal in burn surgery, given the multiple considerations and MDT inputs these patients require. Seniors will expect a high standard of attention to detail. Aim to familiarise yourself with any new admissions and to have the latest results updated.

Table 5.1: Pertinent information when updating the handover list

	Description
Patient Summary	For all patients, include their patient demographics, comorbidities, social history, and dates of injury and of admission. Include a burn demographic, with their location, size (in % TBSA; use rule of 9s), depth and mechanism. Include the type and number of previous operations and the dates of previous surgery. Highlight the current management plan of the patient, including medical, social, surgical and other aspects.
Observations	As discussed in previous chapters, the physiological changes that come with burn injuries can be dramatic. The latest observations should be up to date before the ward round, and they should be interpreted with attention.
Blood Results	There are marked physiological derangements, either secondary to the injury or following interventions, which may or may not need addressing. All patients should have an up-to-date FBC, renal function (acute kidney injury is common, and significantly impacts mortality), liver function, coagulation screen and CRP (marker of infection). An up-to-date group and save, with an appropriate amount of estimated blood loss, should be available for all patients going to theatre.
Microbiology	Burns result in loss of the protective barrier coupled with an immunocompromised state, and patients are at high risk of infection and sepsis. Frequent wound sample and culture with tissue samples or swabs is normal in burns units. Ensure that the latest swab results are in the list, alongside the current antibiotic treatment, its duration and the latest discussion with microbiology.
Other Information	Other key information that needs addressing in the ward round (e.g. medical, psychological or social issues) that may affect clinical management or discharge planning should be briefly summarised in the list.

THE WARD

THE HANDOVER

Patient and theatre lists should be prepared prior to handover. Operative lists should be made available to wards, anaesthetic and theatre staff. Listed cases should include patient and burn demographics with the types of interventions and specific equipment needed. It is not unusual for burns patients to have resistant bacteria, and due to infection prevention concerns, this may impact the order of the list. Thorough operative lists allow the teams to adequately assess and prepare for the cases. Each patient should be consented, operative sites marked, adequately starved, and have all results available to aid the anaesthetic team.

For patients under the care of an intensivist team, information on the patient's clinical status as well as the level of support the patient is receiving should be gathered to adequately discuss the patient at the handover. This often includes ventilatory requirements, ionotropic support, antimicrobial substances, sedation and analgesic requirements, temperature control measures, fluid balance and output control, nutrition support as well results of investigation and observations. This can often be delivered in an A–F fashion (**A**irway, **B**reathing, **C**irculation, neurological **D**isability, **E**xposure, **F**luid).

THE WARD

THE WARD ROUND

Ward rounds on burns units are usually carried out in a standardised format to prevent loss of information and involve members of the MDT. Infection control procedures are paramount and are minimised by changing scrubs, washing hands, limiting patient contact and by the use of barrier protective equipment as appropriate.

During the ward round, review the patient's clinical status (clinical examination of burn, observations, bloods, fluid input/output, pain and medication chart) and correlate this with the current management plans and need for further surgery. Regarding the burn wound, consider the needs of the wound and the dressings required. Part of the discharge for these patients will include the plans from the wider burns MDT, including therapies, and psycho/social needs.

Whilst on the ward and ward round, consider the following:

1. *Pain*: There are objective and subjective measurements of pain and most patients with a burn will require some form of analgesia during their care. Patients should always be consulted and actively managed for their pain. It is not unusual for donor sites to be more painful than the grafted area and the patient should be warned of this preoperatively. Large burns may have psychological needs and anxiety; warning a patient about what to expect during treatment will therefore help reduce perceived pain during procedures. Distraction therapy and play specialists should be used to help children during dressing changes.

   Where patients are not able to express their level of pain, the following may give an idea of a patient's level of pain: respiratory rate, heart rate and volume of sedation. In young children, a scale such as FLACC (**F**ace, **L**egs, **A**rms, **C**ry, **C**onsolability) can be useful. Burns units usually have their own analgesic protocols which should be consulted, and in burns centres there will be burns intensivists who can help. Always consider baseline pain as well as acute events that require analgesia for your patients. Dressing changes, infections and surgical interventions can all affect a patient's analgesia need. Consider supplemental analgesia such as Oramorph®, Entonox® or intranasal diamorphine.

THE WARD

2. *Itching*: This can cause significant discomfort to patients, leading to donor site and wound breakdown. St Andrew's anti-itch ladder, which is specific for burns itches, has four steps that are added as you progress through them: 1) moisturise and cool, 2) gabapentin, 3) cetirizine and cyproheptadine, and 4) chlorphenamine.

3. *Nutrition*: Burn patients require high levels of nutritional support. This is frequently monitored by checking a patient's weight and monitoring albumin levels and trace elements. For all burns patients, you should strive for a positive nitrogen balance. This means the patients can be shifted from a catabolic to an anabolic state. Specific requirements for patient nutrition should always be guided by dietetic support.

4. *Fluid Management*: In acute significant burns, strict fluid balance is necessary to monitor fluid resuscitation, aiming for a urine output of >0.5ml/kg/hr in adults and >1ml/kg/hr in children. Strict care of the catheter is important as this indicates another nidus to infection in patients with a compromised immune system.

5. *Burn Wound Management*: It will be expected that you will know the previous surgical interventions performed, what dressings were applied and when the next change of dressings are expected.

Consideration of Dressing Changes

- Appropriate analgesia needs to be prescribed, as dressing changes can be painful. Some changes will need to be performed in theatres or need sedation with anaesthetic involvement.

- It is important to minimise the time between a dressing being removed and redressed, as this can be painful for the patient and there is a need to minimise potential for infection. This can be done by planning dressing changes in advance, getting the necessary equipment ready beforehand and checking the correct staffing levels are available.

- Any patient who has deteriorated unexpectedly should have their wounds checked, as all burn wounds have a high risk of infection.

THE WARD

POST WARD ROUND

Once the round is completed, all the jobs should be noted clearly and arranged in priority of importance. Detailed notes from the ward round must be kept, discussing all the aspects of patient care we have considered in this chapter. Plans for each patient must be clear and the possibility of discharge made known to the wider team. Once the jobs have been completed and the ward round documented for all patients, the next major task is preparing for the handover. The inpatient and theatre lists should be updated and results from any tests prepped to present. Any urgent outstanding investigation should be made clear to staff to chase for the next shift/on-call team.

THE WARD

DISCHARGE PLANNING

Patient discharges from burns units are always MDT driven and agreed upon. When a patient is medically stable and fit for discharge, many other factors such as psycho-social, family support and home environment need to be considered.

1) Dressings should be manageable in an outpatient environment. Education and support need to be given to patients/parents who may need to perform dressing changes at home.

2) Patients may need ongoing nutritional support, especially large burns or patients with premorbid high alcohol intake.

3) Burns therapy assessment of patient is not just important in hospital but also at home. Home visits by burns therapists may be needed prior to discharge to see if additional packages of care or equipment are needed for the patients to carry out their activities of daily living. For example, a patient with mobility issues may need their bed moving downstairs or need ramps installing to access their home.

4) A patient's place of residence may also not be suitable to return to after a burn injury due to fire damage. This means temporary accommodation may need to be found.

5) Safeguarding can be an issue in both adults and children, which would prevent discharge to their usual residence. Social services, safeguarding and occupational therapists work together to arrange an appropriate, safe discharge with the goal of the patient continuing their recovery in an appropriately safe environment.

6) As burns units are often centralised units with specialty care not found in all hospitals, patients' distance from the hospital needs to be considered. This is especially relevant when patients require multiple complex dressing changes or further surgery post discharge. Transport requirements may lead to financial concerns for the patient and reimbursement may need to be sought from burns charities.

7) There is a high incidence of mental-health illness and drug abuse in burn victims. Psychiatric and psychology teams should have input to assure there is an appropriate outpatient management plan. Psychology input is also required in patients who do not have a known mental-health issue but need psychological support in recovering from a burn injury.

All these variables again point to a heavy reliance on the MDT for the care and discharge of patients from a burns unit.

THE WARD

Final Tips for the Ward Round on a Burns Unit

• Be organised – working on a burns unit can be chaotic. Update the patient list frequently: keeping current plans up to date helps the team recognise where progress is being made or care is plateauing for some patients.

• Always keep track of antibiotic durations on the handover sheet. This will help you point out cases where further microbiological input may be required or treatments stopped.

• Work with the nurses wherever possible. The nursing staff on burns units are highly trained and many have a wealth of knowledge regarding burns. Never be afraid to discuss certain situations with the senior burns nurses. Having a good working relationship with the nursing team will be hugely beneficial as both teams are able to help each other and provide better patient care.

• Knowing your patients' circumstances as well as their clinical state is important. Not having any home support is just as likely to stop a discharge as a missing investigation result. Having this information to relay to your seniors will benefit the team.

THE WARD

INDEX